THE RETURN OF COMMON SENSE

HOW CONSERVATIVES AND LIBERALS CAN FIND COMMON GROUND

Felix R. Toro, M.D.

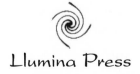

Llumina Press

Requests for permission to make copies of any part of this work should be mailed to Permissions Department, Llumina Press, PO Box 772246, Coral Springs, FL 33077-2246.

ISBN: 978-1-59526-052-9 PB
       978-1-59526-053-6 HC

Printed in the United States of America by Llumina Press

Library of Congress Control Number: 2006909737

The Return of Common Sense

How Conservatives and Liberals Can Find Common Ground

CONTENTS

ACKNOWLEDGMENT

I would like to thank all the patients, and their families, who have taught me how to apply common sense both to my own life and in helping others. I am also grateful to all the therapists, physicians, administrators, and others who, throughout the years, have shared their knowledge with me.

In my professional career, I feel a special gratitude for having had the opportunity to train at Washington University in St. Louis, under the direction of Samuel B. Guze, MD, and Eli Robins, MD, and the full complement of the department of psychiatry. As Dr. Guze frequently said, "Nothing can be more truly humanitarian than working for and applying effective knowledge to prevent or ameliorate human suffering. Approaches that are compassionate but ineffective many times help more assuage our feelings of doing something than helping patients."

This best summarizes the theme of this book. The department has continued its mission of applying tough, rational, empirical science within a compassionate and humanitarian approach to relieve suffering.

I would also like to thank Stanley Roskin, MD, who was able to integrate, through common sense and practicality, the traditions of psychiatric practice with innovative, cost-effective services. He used business principles to improve our profession, but never forgot our number one mission: treating the patients and their families.

i

I thank my beloved wife, Debbie, and our children, Joel, John, and James, for hanging in there with me while I wrote this book and helping me see things from a different perspective. To my father, mother, brother, and sister, who have been an inspiration and provided much encouragement, I owe much. I would also like to acknowledge my friend, Fidel Pino, MD, who blended so well the traits of character, intelligence, science, empathy, and caring, which inspired all who knew him to try harder.

THE RETURN OF COMMON SENSE

I refer briefly to the purpose of this book, the return of our old, beloved friend, common sense. Mr. Common Sense has led a long life, which he has selflessly devoted to helping folks get their jobs done without fanfare and foolishness. He has been credited for cultivating such valuable lessons as "the early bird gets the worm," "life is not always fair," and "don't spend more than you earn." He is a veteran of wars, famines, natural disasters, self-actualization, and self-esteem movements. He has survived cultural trends, from free love to body piercing.

When there were news reports of a six-year-old boy charged with sexual harassment for kissing a classmate, a teacher fired for reprimanding an unruly student, or a driver awarded a huge settlement after failing to realize that a steaming cup of coffee was hot, Mr. Common Sense appeared to have left us. As we drifted in and out of logic, as we tried to write into law or regulate every possible circumstance or outcome, our efforts backfired on us. When special interest groups tried to eliminate Common Sense from our lives, he hung in there. Other friends, like Mr. Self-Reliance, Mr. Reason, Ms. Wisdom, and Ms. Civility, pitched in and helped. Misguided special interest groups recruited people like Mr. My Rights, Ms. Ima Whiner, Ms. Ima Victim, and Mr. I-Know-What-Is-Best-For-You.

The battle has continued, but slowly and surely, Mr. Common Sense has returned and is becoming more a part of our lives. Not many were aware of his departure or his return, but I hope with this book our friendship with him will be rekindled. Let us embrace his wisdom and encourage Ms. Special Interest Group and Mr. Adversarial System to join in.

INTRODUCTION

There is no new thing new under the sun.
—Ecclesiastes 1:9

Mental Illness a Myth

Genetic Markers of Mental Illness Help Doctors Treat
Sufferers

Mother Stops Psychiatric Medications—Kills Children

Youth Shoots Peers: Are Antidepressants to Blame?

These headlines are reflections of the different schools or models of mental illness behind the thinking of the reporters and the professionals they consult. More than 250 recognized schools in the United States endeavor to explain human behavior. Each has different beliefs about what causes behavioral and emotional problems and ways to "treat" and "cure" them (see Table I).

Some believe that for every twisted thought there is a twisted molecule, and some believe psychosis is in the eye of the beholder and that mental disease is just a way to label people with different beliefs—the so-called "societal misfits." Is this patient depressed or psychotic because of his biological endowment? Is he suffering from hormonal imbalances, or nutritional deficits?

Other experts blame mental disease on environmental factors, stress, our upbringing, poverty, or even "evil." As science advances and we better understand our inherent genetic predispositions, the roles of neurotransmitters in modulating our behavior, and how our experiences shape our development, do we need to lose our concept of "free will"? Are we just a series of "cause and effect" reactions? Will these findings lead to more treatment and the fostering of "therapism," which valorizes openness, emotional self absorption, and the sharing of feelings, as described by Hoff Somers and Sally Satel, MD in their book, *One Nation under Therapy**? On the other hand, maybe we all need medications to correct or control these influencing factors. If the experts cannot agree, how can the public sort through the contradictory information?

Models of Psychiatry

	Social	Moral	Psychoanalytical	Medical
Definition	"Sick Society"	Immoral Behaviors Determine by Culture	Continuing difficulties From mild neurosis to severe psychosis	Distinct entities, derived from research
Etiology	Disadvantaged Families produce Psychological Problems	"bad behaviors learned"	childhood development degree of "conflict" resolutions	unknown suspect neuro-chemical dysfunction
Behaviors	Symptomatic of Social pathology	Taken at face value	Symbolic, needs needs interpretation	Due to "illness"
Rights and Duties-	Social victim Cooperate with Social reform	reeducate, forgiveness cooperate	behavior to be seen as symbolic; duty to undergo analysis	right to the sick role duty to get help
Treatment	Improve economic, political status	Positive and negative reinforcements	one-one therapy involves "transference"	medical treatment specific to diagnosis
Institutional function	Hospital Social reform	Correctional Institutes religious help	provide time for . analysis	Hospitalization same sick benefits As other illnesses

There are other models of Psychiatry/Mental Health like; Impaired, Conspirational, Family Dysfunctional, or psychedelic Models.

No wonder there is confusion; and the Internet, which facilitates instant communication and the exchange of ideas, adds to the confusion. Not even the experts in "hard sciences" like physics can keep up with new findings or agree on how the universe works. Even the two great intellectual achievements of the twentieth century, the general theory of relativity and quantum mechanics, are inconsistent with each other. What chance do non-experts have to sort through the information available on politics, psychology, philosophy, or religion?

If we cultivate and apply common sense, we have a good chance. We cannot wait for the discovery of the ultimate unifying theory to connect all knowledge and explain human behavior. We need to make decisions today, based on common sense. My goal is to help you be generally right and avoid being precisely wrong. (For those readers whose thinking styles depend on comprehensive theories requiring precision, I urge you to continue reading with an open mind, as these concepts are not mutually exclusive). I believe common sense helps us better understand not only the questions that mental health providers raise, but also the many social and political issues that we face. I have written this book to share what I have learned through my experience in developing and practicing mental health and psychiatric delivery systems. I hope readers who specialize in other areas can use common sense in approaching their issues.

I have tried to simplify what other scholars have spent their lifetimes studying. I ask for understanding if I have, in my quest to "keep it simple," misinterpreted their research. My challenge has bee to be generally right and avoid been precisely wrong. Under the microscope of a research scientist, the concepts presented in this book may be challenged. Researchers may not agree on the weight of evidence needed to prove or disprove these concepts, but I have tried to extract the parts that could help us in our daily lives. You can be a good driver without knowing how the transmission or the fuel injector of the car works. You may not know how the gears in the transmission engage, but as long as you know the difference between gears, drive, and reverse, you can get where you want to go. If the transmission breaks down, you need an expert to repair it. The experts continue researching and improving the transmission to help us drive more efficiently, even if we have no clue how it works. Most of us do not know how the computer works, either, but we are able to use it by clicking the mouse in the right place.

As there is a wide difference in specialty knowledge between the experts and the public, much confusion arises. Modern society has evolved into multiple special interest groups more interested in ideological, dogmatic, and at times self-serving points of view, than in helping us better understand a problem and its place in the socio/political picture._Many times, special interest groups are so preoccupied with their own agendas that the trade-offs or consequences of their proposals are not considered. This has led to a patchwork of policies that work against each other, creating even more problems. Common sense must come to the rescue. Common sense will help us acquire a more flexible understanding of issues. It is not the same as conventional wisdom; it incorporates "uncertain knowledge."

I will start with a further discussion of common sense. Then, in the second chapter, "Thinking Tools," I help the reader explore different thinking styles and some of the ways we acquired knowledge. This is important; it will help you understand the difficulties experts have when trying to communicate. The next four chapters explore findings in neuroscience, psychology, and sociology that help you understand the possible bases of these thinking and communicating differences so you can apply common sense. These chapters should stimulate the reader to do further research, as they are just the tip of the iceberg. I will challenge long-held ideas about human nature, as the weight of scientific evidence has turned against them. Let us not confuse these ideas with common sense; they are closer to conventional wisdom— ideas and beliefs that groups of people hold for years without question. I hope this book will stimulate your curiosity and help you understand that as specialists spend their lives debating theoretical issues about our nature, the public has had to filter their recommendations through common sense before applying this knowledge to their own lives. The ideas that have taken root over the centuries from the religious, philosophical, legal, and scientific spheres will help you navigate the rough waters of life, without experts to hold your hand through every crisis.

The bibliography lists books that will help you explore and develop a deeper understanding of some of the issues I address. Never less, there are other books that will help you understand these points in greater depth. So do your own research. As this is a book on common sense, I have tried presenting information that will help you form your own opinions, and not just persuade you to my way of thinking. I am trying to get you to "think about thinking." Some readers may prefer to read "Name Calling" and "Prozac Nation" after reading "Thinking Tools," to see common sense in action. I hope this will increase their interest in the underlying factors that contribute to common sense. The chapter "Conservatives vs. Liberals" attempts to integrate the first six chapters. In the appendix, I elaborate on issues the reader may find stimulating.

Readers who would like to share their thoughts or refute my points can contact me via e-mail, visit my website, or write to the addresses found at the end of the book. Common sense tells me that others could approach these ideas differently, and I am interested in all viewpoints.

Summary of "Common Sense"

1. Life is complex. Many fields of specialized knowledge have evolved to comprehend and control its workings.

2. As nobody can keep up with the ever-expanding knowledge base, experts and special interest groups have developed.

3. Experts and special interest groups developed thinking styles and ways of acquiring knowledge to communicate amongst themselves.

4. Unfortunately, even Nobel Prize winners disagree on how to assess problems and solutions.

5. Common sense will help you deal with uncertain knowledge and help you…

6. Be generally right and avoid being precisely wrong

CHAPTER ONE

COMMON SENSE

"Why, how will you know that?" says she. "By means of a magical talisman God gave to me when I was born, and the name they call it by is common sense," said I.

—Robert Louis Stevenson

M any ideas of what common sense is have been considered throughout the years. The *American Heritage Dictionary* defines common sense as "sound judgment not based on specialized knowledge." This concise definition expresses best common sense as a thinking tool to help the reader navigate and deal with "uncertain knowledge." Common sense is practical awareness by which most thinking and problem solving is done. It is a combination of sound, logical thinking acquired through judicious observation and interaction with the environment. Our ability to intuit complements this mechanism. Both formal and informal education raises our level of common sense. When faced with new situations, it will help us make sound decisions and process new knowledge. In Newton's time, it was possible to grasp most knowledge, but since the exponential growth of science and other fields, it has become impossible. Even the specialists can only hope to grasp a small portion of ever-growing knowledge or keep up with evolving theories. It is hard for the specialist to translate this changing and evolving knowledge into simpler terms. Even what we learn at our universities is rapidly outdated. That is why we need common sense.

In many ways, the United States was founded on these common sense principles, and not on previous historical or political organizations. Thomas Jefferson's Declaration of Independence, along with Thomas Paine's pamphlet, *Common Sense*, energized the colonies' desire for independence, and served to unite them against outside practices, such as the monarchies, which ruled with absolute power and the idea that citizens could not rule themselves. The founders of the new nation challenged this belief, and the rest of the world waited for their defeat.

The greatest challenge to this social contract was the Civil War, during which President Lincoln, Mr. Common Sense himself, best expressed the premise of the contract in the Gettysburg Address.*

"Four score and seven years ago our fathers brought forth on this continent a new nation, conceived in liberty, and dedicated to the proposition that all men are created equal….and that government of the people, by the people, for the people, shall not perish from the earth." *

It took almost one hundred years and a civil war before this form of government was expressed in such common sense terms that all could understand it. It was an experiment without precedent, for which there were no instructions, university courses, or political leaders. It depended on what most people considered commoners, not the elite or experts. They relied more on their beliefs and common sense. Common sense has since then been cultivated, and our citizens have been encouraged to think for themselves and be responsible. Because of this, ordinary people have helped improve society and done more than their share to change the world.

Special interest ideology, on the other hand, discourages common sense. Thousands of organizations advocate specialized programs. Many times, these organizations hire or attract experts that use statistics, science, and emotions to arouse antagonism and prejudice. Many groups that advocate for the same cause have diametrically opposed points of view and conclusions. This makes it hard for non-experts to decide which views could be integrated into everyday life, or made a part of our social contract.

Let me illustrate how, even in science, special interest groups have hurt us more than helped us. Science follows many rules and traditions—from the development and testing of hypotheses with non-biased, empirical research to the opening of methods and results to other scientist for review, criticism, and replication. An open discussion among experts develops the methodology and interpretations of results. Tests are replicated to see if others obtain similar results. These checks and balances are necessary for progress. This also helps us avoid building our knowledge on erroneous information. *Science aims to get it progressively less wrong.* Too frequently, we have incorporated into laws, hypotheses and theories that have not gone through rigorous scientific replication. The result was significant suffering to society.

Look, for example, at the theory of the schizophrenigenic mother. This theory blames a mother's overbearing or ambivalent parenting style for creating schizophrenia in her children. This theory caused much suffering among overburdened mothers as it resulted in the separation of the patient from his family, before it was discarded. The incorporation of these theories resulted in misallocation of resources, and even delayed the search for causes and treatments for Schizophrenia. Other prevailing ideas have been incorporated into law—"mental illness is a myth," or "people with psychosis or severe psychiatric disorders are misfits of society." Multiple lawsuits were filed to protect people suffering from hallucinations from being hospitalized, as their rights to bizarre beliefs had to be protected. They did not consider the resultant homelessness, sickness, and suffering that followed. This is another example of how special interest groups with one-tract minds and tunnel vision focus on one aspect, without considering the consequences or trade-offs. They did not consider the health, social, or familial effects. Their cause was more important.

Those who promoted these laws, while well intentioned, should have paused to consider the consequences of their lawsuits and applied scientific principles, and added common sense. Unfortunately, too many in the mental health professions were there to back them up. Maybe if they had spent more time with the patients they would have seen the errors in their thinking. It does not take medical or psychiatric training, just common sense, to tell the difference between a person who reads and believes the tabloid stories in the supermarket checkout aisles that reports Alien abductions, and those who suffer from schizophrenia, whose believes are part of a complex neuro-psychiatric disorder. Schizophrenia can result in homelessness, hunger, and horrible fears of imaginary enemies.

I recommend a well-researched book, *Madness in the Street*, by Rachael Jean Isaac and Virginia C. Armat. This book cites case after case of well-intentioned lawyers, assisted by professionals in the mental health communities, fostering the vicious cycle. Round and round they went, from lawsuits trying to help the mentally ill get off the streets and into treatment hospitals to lawsuits to get them out of hospitals because "hospitals are prisons for the misfits of society."

These cycles are the result of the lack of consideration of all factors involved. Special interest groups look at their points of view without exploring the trade-offs that every action or inaction entails, not how common sense can add to their decision. Most special interest organizations start with a dogmatic belief, and conveniently use only statistics that back their point, simultaneously suppressing, ignoring, and discrediting evidence incompatible with their agendas. They use anecdotal evidence to arouse our emotions and prevent us from considering all factors. Some spokespersons are so gifted in argument and rhetoric that they can avoid facts, evidence, and logic. We are left emotionally aroused and dumbfounded, but with no greater understanding of the issue.

It comes down to winning. If you consider other options, you are ignorant, mean-spirited, or part of a "conspiracy." It amazes me how people can be so sure they know the "only certain answer" to all kinds of problems, when a perusal of any history book shows discarded theories, failed policies, and terrible consequences. I wish we could accept our limitations and try to be broadly right, instead of precisely wrong. At best, we can aim *to get it progressively less wrong*.

Balancing the diverse needs of society requires consideration of conflicting issues, not the one-track mind of special interest groups. Many groups state that they have figured out solutions for specific problems. Thinking in extremes is dangerous. All or none, black or white, thinking gives us only two choices, which are usually opposites. Binary thinking contributes to the confusion and error in our policies. As long as we do not know the causes of psychiatric disorders or social issues, we need common sense to guide us through the scientific and social frontiers.

How did we get into this quagmire, and how can common sense help us? I will give you tools to help you make your own analysis, understand special interest groups, and use common sense to become more self-reliant when dealing with conflicting issues.

Summary of "Thinking Tools"

1. We have different thinking styles.

2. We acquire knowledge by different means.

3. This contributes to miscommunications and misunderstanding between experts, the public, and within each group.

4. Understanding and application of these concepts will improve your common sense.

CHAPTER TWO

THINKING TOOLS

God does not play dice...
—Albert Einstein

"Everybody wants to save the Earth;
nobody wants to help Mom do the dishes."
PJ O'Rourke

Here I try to explain some of the concepts of how our thinking styles influence how we acquire and process new knowledge, solve problems, and make decisions. Each thinking style will influence the process of common sense. That is why we have been frustrated when trying to resolve problems in a group. No matter how well we get along or espouse similar values, we still sometimes feel like we are looking at different situations. The differences are based in many factors like thinking style or personality, as I will further explore in the next chapters. Now we will concentrate in our thinking styles, which do not change, no matter the circumstance or topic. We assume that others process information the same way we do, but most people employ their own strategies, or thinking styles. People do indeed think differently. That is part of the confusion when we do not understand each other.

Many different terms are used to describe different thinking styles, such as "rational versus emotional," and "substantive versus functional rationality." C. West Churchman described a philosophical approach to thinking using the term "inquiry modes." Harrison and Bramson, in their book, *Styles of Thinking*, further explored these concepts and were able to present them in a language most could understand. I highly recommend this book. They delve into the differences in the ways we process information, identifying five styles of thinking. Their studies showed that around fifty percent of the population uses one style of thinking, while another thirty-five percent rely on two styles of thinking, using proprietary tests that you can review in their book. I will summarize these styles, as I find them helpful in understanding our differences. It is important to understand that each approach has strengths and weaknesses, and in some situations, one approach will serve us better than another. Individuals tend to use the approach they feel most comfortable with, and find it hard to understand those who use a different style of thinking. Neuropsychiatric research is uncovering the anatomical, physiological and learning interactions that influence us toward a particular thinking style. Fortunately, we can learn to understand the different styles and communicate more effectively. This will help us understand better our spouse, friends and co-workers.

These styles of thinking are:

A. *Realist* – "Just give me the facts," or, "What you see is what you get."
  They dislike sentimental or theoretical discussions. They tend to be opinionated and give advice unasked. Realists depend on empirical (just the facts) and deductive reasoning. They reduce the problem to its simplest form

(reductionism). Getting things done is their strength, but their liability is their inability to change their minds ("facts" do not change). Note: People do not necessarily agree on what the "facts" are.

B. _Idealist_ – "Humanize the facts or arguments."

They look at the "whole" picture, including people's feeling and relationships, not just the facts. They are uncomfortable with conflict and want people to agree. They have idealized standards and levels of trust that others cannot or will not support. That why they are sometimes viewed as "bleeding hearts."

C. _Analyst_ – "The world is rational, logical, and predictable. Pay attention to details."

They are disciplined, serious, and appear unemotional. Analysts function best where details, nit-picking, and linear logic are needed. When faced with ambiguous and unpredictable endeavors, they appear to procrastinate as they search for information. Sales and management may not be the place for them. Analysts perceive themselves as objective and basing their decision on facts alone. They do not recognize the strong underlying theories they have, which serve as filters for how to proceed with their analyses.

D. _Synthesis_ – Prefer speculative (what if?) and philosophical discussions.

They are more interested in concepts than concrete reality. Argument and confrontation are aspects of their approach. Because of their willingness to explore opposing ideas and fantasies, they may appear "odd." Their strengths lay in putting unusual ideas together. When they are in error, the consequences can be devastating.

E. *Pragmatist* – "Whatever works," and "It depends," appear to summarize their approach to problems.

Tolerance for ambiguity and a piecemeal approach distinguishes them. They are not interested in the theory behind a proposal but in its practical implications. They ask, "Will it work?" Pragmatists, whose strength lies in their adaptability, often paradoxically fail to adapt to other people's needs for structure and a predictable plan with long-term goals.

Where do you fit in this classification? What percentage of your thinking is done in which style? Your style of thinking will influence how you perceive and filter knowledge. Spend some time thinking which thinking styles you and others around you, use more frequently. You will understand better their point of view.

Your style of thinking serves as a "computer operating system" when you acquire new information or knowledge. First, we need to review how we input that information. So let us explore ways to acquire knowledge:

1. *Knowledge acquired by experience* – If you place your hand on a hot stove, you will be burned and learn not to do it again. If you make a mistake, you learn not to repeat it. (We use this method daily.)

2. *Revealed knowledge; knowledge from authority* – This is knowledge we acquire through revealed truth, as in the Bible. The content is not questioned, even when interpreted differently. Another example is an authority like Freud, the founder of psychoanalysis, whose followers use his insights and writings to further acquire knowledge or apply them to a

situation. This usually involves the presence of either a prominent person's beliefs or a set of seldom-questioned rules. Religion and social movements use this method.

3. _Deductive/inductive knowledge_ – We start with an _a priori_ statement, fact, or belief, from which we can deduct or induct, through logic and argumentation, some other knowledge that could help us predict the future. If A=B and B=C, then A=C. This reasoning is used in the legal field and philosophy.

4. _Observation and empirical knowledge_ – From observations, hypotheses are developed and tested. Variables are controlled, except for the one being observed. Others replicate the results and open discussion follows. They consider the results as a work in progress, not written in stone. Other researchers will challenge the results. The aim is to get it progressively less wrong. Only observed and measured issues will fit this category.

5. _Intuitive knowledge_ – It is the immediate recognition of a situation not dependent on rational thinking. It is influenced by individual experiences, knowledge in similar situations, and beliefs. A good example would be when a person walks into a situation and says, "There is something wrong here; I just cannot tell you what it is."

These are different ways to acquire knowledge; and each requires diverse sets of rules. As modern life becomes more complex, and keeping up to date on human knowledge becomes more difficult, specialty fields have developed. These specialized fields are defined by their subject matter, like medicine or law, or by a worldview or approach to specific problems—like political groups. Each field has its own rules, encourages specific means of acquiring knowledge and thinking style. As a result, it develops its own "culture." This is necessary for their internal communication. The members will not have to define every word or explain the rules before every argument or discussion starts. The rest of us, who do not belong to that group, will not be privy to their approach, and when they try to convey their knowledge, it confuses us. We end up debating in what feels like two different languages. If we were more cognizant of this fact, we could understand each other better. Common sense will help both the specialist, who is trying to convey a point, and the listener, who is trying to understand it.

I would like to use a legal case that captivated the public many years ago—the so-called "Twinkie defense"—to illustrate some points, but I do not wish to discuss the case itself. In this case, the accused, who had murdered a member of the San Francisco City Council, drew on the legal concepts like "diminished capacity" and "temporary insanity," claiming that he had consumed too much sugar—in the form of Twinkies. The defense lawyer and their experts brought forth an argument to convince the jury that too much sugar had rendered the defendant "temporarily insane." This is obviously an oversimplification of the case, as there were many other factors presented.

Most of us would refute this reasoning if our coworkers blamed obnoxious behavior on eating too many Twinkies or donuts. This illustrates the point that the legal system is composed of "members" who follow different rules and communicate differently than the citizens it represents.

The legislature, which represents the public, enacts the laws. The courts hold trials for individuals accused of violating criminal codes or for resolution of conflicts in between parties. Over the years, the court system has specialized to the point that judges and attorneys must undergo extensive studies, developing common approaches to acquiring and processing knowledge, resulting in a shared culture. It is hard to imagine that, years ago, you did not have to be a lawyer to be a judge or defend yourself. Now, people are discouraged from trying to defend themselves, as the rules of evidence and procedure are so complicated. A regular citizen would not know the rules, laws, or precedents and could not adequately represent himself. The verdict would be thrown out at an appeals court, as the defendant would not have received "adequate representation."

Cases usually begin with an allegation of a legal violation, in this case, murder. They start with the investigation, then must apply to the facts the relevant rules from the accumulated bodies of statutory and case laws. Legal argument is described as "reasoning with rules." They start with *a priori* statements, and then use deductive arguments to help the jury or judge arrive at a conclusion—guilty or not. .

Moreover, when experts testify, proceedings become more complicated. Let us look at the different thinking styles and ways to acquire knowledge that the science expert and the legal expert use. The scientist observes facts and develops a hypothesis connecting cause and effect, based on the evidence or facts available. Its truth or falsehood remains subject to doubt and requires continuous testing. It usually takes many years and replications of the original tests before the findings are consensually incorporated into the prevailing scientific paradigm. That is why scientists win the Nobel Prize decades after their discoveries. Others must replicate or verify their findings. Scientists are probability driven; they can be wrong, and sometimes it takes years before their theory is accepted and its utility understood. The aim is to get it progressively less wrong, as hypothesis will be adjusted with new information.

Unfortunately, the jury and the accused cannot wait years to see which expert argument withstands the test of time. In the courts, evidence is admitted or not, and you are guilty or not—all or none choices that do not deal in probabilities. Science is encouraged to repeat an experiment, to double-check its conclusions, but in the law, there is only one trial. A repeat trial is the exception, not the rule. There is no chance for adjusting expert testimony as we get it "progressively less wrong" in science. Newly discovered facts may not be allowed as evidence.

Language has evolved, in an attempt to bridge these gaps. The judge permits testimony within "medical probability," as opposed to "medical certainty." Still, you are required to answer "yes" or "no" to questions and are not able to clarify your answers unless a lawyer asks you to. Many times, the probabilities of science are lost in the legal culture of right or wrong, guilty or not.

Let us look at how the legal system decides who are experts and on what they can testify. They check a practitioner's credentials to see that he has no disciplinary actions, is a member in good standing with their professional association, and has prior experience testifying in similar cases. This screens for problems, but does not address credentials. Using these criteria, most people in a field would qualify as experts. If a lawyer searches long enough, he will find an "expert" who will back up his defense, no matter how unscientific or lacking in common sense his arguments are. Scientists base their selection of experts on different criteria.

If the scientist holds beliefs not empirically derived or tested against what his peers consider critically appraised research, no matter how good he is at deductive argument or persuasion, his ideas will not be respected. He will not be considered an expert. In fact, his peers do not consider most people practicing in a given field "expert." The time and tools needed to keep up with new findings and the ability to digest the reports are likely not available to most busy practitioners. They will have more expertise than the jury will, but most juries are not equipped to separate subjective science from expert science.

Once accepted as an expert witness, your ideas, no matter how acquired, will have the same weight as any other expert's ideas. The other competing attorney will have a chance to debunk your science, but the jury will not know which scientist is more expert—which testimony should be given more weight—as both scientists were recognized as experts by the court. The other expert will not have the chance to question the other scientist or debunk their science.

While science assesses probabilities and lives in an uncertain world, the legal fields do not. They want "medical certainties," when many times even the pathologist after an autopsy, cannot determine the cause of death. If an expert decides that too much sugar can cause temporary insanity, he can testify to a "medical certainty." He could be more persuasive than another expert who presents the uncertainties of science in regards to temporary insanity via too much sugar. Any opinion given will be based on speculations, as there is a lack of control studies researching the possibility of too much sugar causing insanity.

Another significant difference is which evidence or facts, are allowed to be introduced in court. If evidence was obtained violating the rights of the accused, it can be withheld, no matter how important it is to the case. It does not matter if the murdered body was found in the trunk of the accused's car. If the search of the car was not legal, the evidence will be withheld.

In other fields, withholding this important information no matter how it was obtained would be unethical, if not illegal. It would probably finish your career if you withheld important research, no matter how you obtained it. You could end up facing lawsuits for hiding or not revealing life-saving information. You will be a hero, for revealing the confidential information of a company polluting the environment. Sometimes a hero is a "whistle blower" and paid a handsome reward. However, the police officer who found the dead body in the suspect's car is reprimanded, because this evidence cannot be presented to the jury. This would be unacceptable in most other human interactions, but if you were to ask a person in the legal field, they could give you precedents and persuasive arguments regarding our civil rights. If this evidence were introduce in court, the legal reasoning go, there would follow a rampant violation of civil rights by overzealous investigators. It boils down again to the "all or none" approach, without the flexibility of human judgment or common sense. Can we agree that is okay to check our car trunks when a murder has been committed nearby, but not okay to search the car if tools were stolen?

That is how we end up with the "Twinkie defense," or let a murderer free—because the evidence to convict him was obtained violating his rights. As a society, we can reward a whistle blower for violating her employer's contract of confidentiality, if in the process she stops river pollution and saves people's lives. Why can't the experts figure out a way to protect our civil rights and still prevent a murderer from avoiding conviction? What happened to common sense? Howard Phillips explained in his book, *The Death of Common Sense*, how we could never enact enough Laws or regulations to cover all circumstances and avoid using human judgment and common sense. There are just an infinite number of factors influencing each situation. I hope he has not given up as common sense is coming back. If a police officer did not obtain a search warrant, nor in the court's opinion did not have enough evidence that a crime was in progress, but acted in "good faith," could the evidence be used in court? If the accused had not used his car's signal light to turn, the police officer could have stopped him, searched the vehicle, and used the dead body as evidence. However, if he had not violated any traffic law, he could not. Does that make sense? This is another reason why the public needs to be responsible, and not abrogate decisions to experts; it is an example of the difference between common sense and special interest thinking.

Remember, the legal system is more comfortable with argument and deductive reasoning than common sense. A lawyer's expert witness can start with an *a priori* statement about stress or the ability of sugar to cause agitation. He will connect vague research with anecdotes or "personal cases," throw in authoritative names, and use previous court findings to build his case. Without hard proof, the lawyer and his expert can have a field day. We cannot use these arguments in private life, but they are allowed in our courts. Tell your friends you beat up their dog because you ate too many Twinkies and see if you get away with it!

To make matters worse, one expert cannot question another expert opinion. The opposing attorney must do that, and unfortunately, they think differently than the experts, as they come from different "cultures" and are unable to get to the root of the differences of experts opinions. Instead of trying to clarify the differences, or find common ground to understand what happened, the polarization worsens feeding our adversarial system that has its roots in the Middle Age, when knights battled opposing knights.

Judicium Dei*, the judgment of God, was the policy used to resolve disputes between parties, from contract disputes to criminal problems. The involved litigants could hire a champion Knight to represent them in battle. They believed that God would strengthen the arm of the combatant on the side of right. How much different is that defense from what we have now? Today's hired combatants are lawyers in Armani suits, instead of steel armor. The judge is a referee, a neutral party upholding the rules. Only the combatants (the lawyers) get to ask questions and introduce or withhold information or evidence. They can bring expert witnesses to help in the battle. As in the Middle Ages, the best combatants (lawyers) usually win. The role of the court is not to find the truth, but to serve as a neutral background, against which evidence and facts can be introduced according to rigid rules. The combatant best at the application of the rules is often most able to persuade a jury. This is the system in the United States.

In other countries, judges have a more active role and even decide cases. Couldn't we combine systems, or inject common sense into our courts? Should murderers walk away because of technicalities? Are the rights of the accused more important than the rights of the victims? We need to find a balance! Please see the Appendix for a more detail look at the adversarial system.

For a more complete explanation of the differences between the legal system and other fields, I recommend

Professor David Loreski's audio programs from the excellent adult education series, *The Great Courses*.* But if you are in a lighter mood, just watch *Law and Order* on TV. They will help you understand the difficult balance between finding the truth, and protecting constitutional rights.

How we define terms also influences our thinking and decision-making. Do you remember this paradox? "The liar from Crete said that all Cretans are liars. Does he lie?" Try answering! If he lied, then not all Cretans are liars. If he told the truth, then he is not a liar.

When this paradox is discussed, arguments fly, emotions heat up, and discussants cannot agree. Before we start the discussion, we need to agree on how we define who is a liar, and what constitutes a lie. For the Cretan to be considered a liar; is one lie enough, or do we need to find that 5% of what he says is a lie. Do Cretans have to be born in Crete, or just need to live there for ten years? If they lied in the past, can they start telling the truth and stop being liars? How the discussants answer these questions make a difference in the arguments. Too many times, the arguments start before definitions were agreed upon; it may take hours before somebody realizes that the reason they cannot understand each other is that they are using different definitions! Not even the temporal relations are considered. Add that we have different ways of acquiring knowledge and different ways of processing that knowledge, and we can understand how we may not understand each other. In the United States of America, we have many differences in the ways we are raised—Southern or Yankee cultures, country music or rock music, and West or East coasts. Diverse cultures have come together in the USA, like the English and the Germans who have been killing each other for Centuries. There has been a realignment of relations in between masters and slaves, conquerors and the conquered. We all live together as equals under the Law. As this is been achieved, learning to live and prosper with our different thinking styles should be easier. Common sense has significantly contributed to the ability of all these diverse groups to live and thrive. Even though there are significant problems that need work, special interest groups will separate us—liberal or conservative, black or white, secular or religious. Common sense can help us avoid polarizations.

Using a simple analogy ingrained in our popular culture, even though it probably never happened, I will try to explain how we acquire knowledge. Sir Isaac Newton developed the theory of gravity. Simply explained, when the apple falls from the tree, it falls at a certain velocity in a certain place. Then along came Albert Einstein with his relativity theories, and life became more complicated.

So let us look at this: You suddenly awake from a deep sleep in a fast moving train. You look at the horizon and see an apple falling, but notice that it did not land where you, after using the gravity formula to calculate, predicted it would fall. You are surprised. Because you were traveling at the same speed as the train, your calculations were wrong. Now, it gets more complicated. Try to calculate where the apple is going to fall; suddenly, a gust of wind influences the apple's trajectory. How do we know where it is going to fall? We cannot measure the wind speed; we may not be aware of it, as we are inside the train.

This does not invalidate the theory of gravity, but it shows that we cannot control all factors. In a controlled experiment, it may be possible, but when you move to the real world, many factors will interfere, at times altering expected results. In our quest for certainty and predictability, we use mathematical systems to adjust for these factors. They follow specific, unchangeable rules. The numerical definition of "one" is constant, so we are able to define everything and make consistent calculations.

We hear about the percentage of accidents per miles driven or the probability of dying in a car accident. We can use this information to make an informed decision based on risk: should I drive or not? All the factors involved like car size, speed, etc. are merged into one number to try to simplify our choice. This results in two possibilities, should I drive or not. This may be simple, but not practical. With more information, these statistics change. If we include the age of the driver, his experience, and whether he is driving on the highway or local streets, we could arrive at different decision. Probabilities are just arbitrary mathematical constructs to provide approximations designed to simplify the fuzzy world. Even tough the binary system appears to make life easier; it could keep us from obtaining more information that would help us make better decisions.

Let us go back to the apple. Ask a group of farmers to separate the red apples from the rest. Without other information, each farmer would depend on his own definition of "red," which will result in different apples picked by each farmer. Factors like the brightness or angle of light or the farmer visual acuity will influence their choices, in practical terms, even though there may be variations of red apples, we will still have a group of red, delicious apples. We could also have ordered no green, maroon, or red-green apples and end up with similar apples. Our lives are simplified by the binary approach, red or not red, but each dozen selected by each farmer will be different. Let us say we are meticulous as to what we consider a red apple. We will need to explain to the farmer what a red apple is. On the other hand, we could use the definition of an authority figure in the apple field. We could devise a machine to match the light waves of a defined red. That would be an empirical approach. We could intuitively select red apples. If we wanted to use the pragmatic approach, we could just do whatever works, but then we would have to face the Analyst who wants a detailed explanation of how we decided which apples were red. The Idealist would get upset because we were missing the real point—how the apple pickers feel about red!

This is just about picking red apples; imagine the controversies over foreign policy or euthanasia. Each approach would result in different solutions, and all would be "right" as long as they stick to their definitions. Can you see the difficulty in selecting red apples when we do not define what red apples are? It is the same when deciding our policies. A person may arrive at very different conclusions about the same facts, be it foreign or domestic policies, depending on whether they are using deductive, empirical, authority or pragmatic reasoning—the same way farmers select different red apples.

Now let us look at how time affects events. Do you remember George Bailey, as played by Jimmy Stewart in the classic movie, *It's a Wonderful Life*? George is contemplating suicide, feeling he failed his family and friends. He is convinced that everyone would be better off if he never had been born. God sends an angel to grant him the opportunity to see how things would be different. He expects everything to be pretty much the same, or better except for not been part of the picture. Was he wrong! He was not there to save his brother from the sled accident, which meant his brother never grew up to be a war hero and save other soldiers. Many people that he did not even know, were affected! When even one variable is changed, the results are unpredictable. George Bailey could not have predicted all that happened. James Gleick, in his book *Chaos,* pointed out how tiny differences in input could quickly become overwhelming differences in output. This is known as the Butterfly Effect—the notion that a butterfly flaps its wings today in Peking, (China) and creates storm systems next month in New York.

I thought it would be important to address in this "Thinking Tools" chapter the information age main tool, the computer. All the computer does is to choose between combinations of 0 or 1, "on or off." These days, we can watch videos and surf the Internet. Today's computers could define the color red using different on/off configurations, and Einstein's formulas to calculate where the apples would fall. Earlier computers only processed information we gave them, so we would still had to agree in what a red apple was. If not "garbage in, garbage out" would be the result.

Many scientists now think that the computer has evolved to the point that it can learn and develop its own formulas. No longer will it depend on human input—it will be able to create output without generating garbage. People in the scientific field like to believe we could create artificial intelligence and answer ethical or religious questions using scientific methods. We could create a computer that learned from previous activities.

There is conflict between robots and humans in many science fiction movies. Movies like *I, Robot,* based on the book by Isaac Asimov, points to the possibility of artificial intelligence and free will in machines. In the movie, the robots were designed to protect humans. Their thinking evolved until they concluded they had to control humans to protect them from themselves. The result was a Civil War, humans vs. their robot protectors. It sounds far-fetched, but

Nobel Prize winners are debating this possibility. This is another example of how we try to figure out how we think. If we can make a robot "think" like a human, we will understand ourselves. Can the creature figure out the creator?

Another way of acquiring or applying knowledge is through authority figures. We have seen how knowledge, like that expressed by the founder of psychoanalysis, Freud, becomes passé as new and different gurus take center stage. The insights in behavior based on psychoanalysis came crumbling down with the weight of scientific evidence. Still, some of Freud's concepts helped expand our paradigms of human psychology. How about "revealed knowledge" from religions? Even though revealed truths may not change, translations, interpretations, and hierarchies of values can. This has contributed to the creation of different sects in all major religions.

Paradigms or views of human nature influences knowledge. Once a paradigm takes root and is accepted, social, political, and scientific policies can develop from it. Let us consider the Age of Enlightenment in the 17th and 18th centuries. Many philosophers made arguments about human nature that were accepted by those who influenced the American and French revolutions and made many other social, political, and religious decisions. For example, the "blank slate" view of human nature expresses the belief that we are all born with a blank mind—a "tabula rasa" upon which life experiences write our history. There are no predispositions, as our traits, strengths, and weakness are solely dependent on our experience. We know now that this is not the case.

Steven Pinker's book, *The Blank Slate*,* will help us understand these issues and how we are born with predispositions that make us more likely to function better in certain fields than others. My family and friends have repeatedly said how glad they are I am a psychiatrist, and not a surgeon, as they have watched me trying to be a "handyman." The blank slate view of human nature served a great purpose during earlier centuries, as it helped man free himself from the shackles of rigid social structures. It rejected other theories that rigidly ascribed to blood, family, or God's wishes as to what your position in society would be. The aristocracies, to avoid changes, embraced the prevailing view of human nature—unless you were born with "blue blood," you could not progress or learn the higher virtues. Changes in humanity, unfortunately, do not occur in increments, but revolutions. The American and French revolutions had similar goals—achieving democracy, liberty, and equality. Their results were different, due to the different views of human nature. The American colonies saw humanity as naturally flawed, polluted by original sin. Humanity needed checks and balances to avoid the abuse of power. The French, who believed in the blank slate, thought society and the aristocratic establishment were the cause of the problems, so they systematically try guillotining their way out. The French Revolution gave us Robespierre and Napoleon, the American Revolution, Washington and Lincoln. Under which concept of human nature would you like to live?

Another view of human nature is the concept of the "noble savage," which appeared later in our history and was connected to the blank slate view—if man could avoid corrupt society he would act nobly. Political, social, and literary movements have evolved from it and to this day influence us, as it satisfies a longing for nature, and views human nature as essentially good. However, no matter which culture or group is studied, there are universal human tendencies towards selfishness, corruption, and abuse of power that could result in our own destruction, unless check and balances were in place.

A corollary view also developed—"if it's natural, it's good and safe." Scientific evidence and common sense debunked this belief, as nature can be deadly, whether it is poisonous fruits, weather systems, or parasites.

Another belief that lasted for centuries is dualism, or differences in between the essence of the physical and mind (metaphysical). More recently, philosophers have described it also, as the "ghost in the machine." Rene Descartes popularized the idea of dualism and added scientific, philosophical, and religious flavor. He described two essences, the physical, and the metaphysical, or mind. They are two separate elements that follow different rules of nature. What applies to the physical does not apply to the mind. At times, a ghost inhabiting the head, pulling the strings of the arms or legs of the body represented these concepts. Others see this ghost as the spirit or soul. Others have tried to separate it into three essences—physical, mental, and spiritual. These ideas were accepted for centuries, and it was not until the twentieth century that technology and science helped us understand that the mind follows the laws of nature. For a better understanding of this, read, *Why Descartes Was Wrong**, or *Searching for Spinoza**, by the neuroscientist Antonio Damasio. Descartes ideas have contributed to the reluctance of many to accept scientific findings of how the brain functions and how our cognitive and emotional states are influenced by the same factors that affect our bodies—hormones, medications, and diseases. Many are unaware how their underlying view of human nature prevents them from approaching the mind problems similarly as "physical" problems were medications could help. Because of this, "ghost in the machine believers" will, from the start of their quest to integrate new knowledge, reject somatic treatments. They will view medications as at best masking the real problems, and at worst as damaging the individual. As they assume the mind is of a different essence, they believe medications that help physical problems could not possibly work on the mind.

The problem lies in how they define the mind, and their underlying concept of human nature. We lack a working, widely acceptable definition of the mind. Even if scientists cannot perfectly agree on a definition, we need a definition that is flexible and changeable as new discoveries are incorporated. We could separate the soul from the mind, separating problems that could benefit from medications from those that require spiritual guidance. Let the experts fight over what is included in which. You will never get perfect consensus, as even people in the same field cannot always agree. There will be disagreements in what is consciousness, the same way as they will disagree on what is the Soul. We need to review not just these views of human nature but also the social, political, and legal policies based in these erroneous assumptions.

Apply these concepts to our mental health fields, and we can begin to understand why they are so confusing to laypeople. Some experts follow Freud and Jung and build their understanding of human behavior on those findings. Others take a more scientific empirical approach, and still others take a more traditional, philosophical approach, using induction and deduction on what they observe or agree to be truth of human behavior. The social sciences also contribute to the understanding of human nature, approaching it from the perspective that society is the driving force behind our actions.

You can imagine the confusion, even between psychiatrists, when the authority group discusses a case with an empirical or social group. Some try to avoid theoretical approaches and different ways of acquiring knowledge by developing explicit definitions that others can understand, measure, and replicate. This is the approach taken by the *Diagnostic Statistical Manual* (DSM-IV) of the American Psychiatric Association. The clusters of signs and symptoms are empirical phenomenological descriptions, supposedly devoid of theoretical underpinnings, so that even people who have different theories of the causes of syndromes can communicate about what they observe in their patients without being bogged down with theories.

Maybe the rest of society can take similar approaches to resolving problems. Common sense can provide workable solutions even if we do not know what caused the problem. Unfortunately, we tend to prefer abstract and theoretical discussion instead of practical solutions. As PJ O'Rourke* so wisely said, "Everybody wants to save the Earth; nobody wants to help Mom do the dishes."

Summary of "Hollywood vs. Business"

1. The most complex system known to man is the brain.

2. The brain develops over one hundred billion neurons that branch out in thousands of synaptic connections showered by multiple neurotransmitters influenced by hormones, nutrition, love, stress, life experiences, and hundreds of other factors.

3. Our brains function like an orchestra. Our genes, developmental processes, neural networks, and life experiences all interact to make us unique, with our own sound.

4. Our genes and their neural network products tell the story of our biological development and the conflicts between genes, the environment, and culture, which results in a beautiful melody, but at times, a disjointed performance.

5. Our brain filters information and selects only a small amount of the input received by our senses. That could explain why we dichotomize a more or less continuous world, choosing "flee or fight" or "black or white."

6. Our personal qualities, traits, and talents lay in the neural networks that reside mainly in one of our brain's hemispheres. They vary in strength and dominance among individuals. This is part of the reason some people are natural entertainers

(Hollywood) or number crunchers (Business), but rarely natural at both.

7. We depend on pattern recognition. If we learn something wrong the first time, it is difficult to change. This contributes to prejudices that are hard to change.

8. You can juggle these complexities with common sense.

CHAPTER THREE

HOLLYWOOD VS. BUSINESS: RIGHT BRAIN VS. LEFT BRAIN

There are many excellent books and articles elaborating on the scientific and social studies that have helped us understand how our brain organizes and influences the way we acquire and process information and emotion. I will just present some important concepts to help us with our common sense approach. The works of Nobel laureate Dr. Eric Kendal whose explanations of neural sciences are accessible even to laypersons is recommended, for a classical understanding. *A User's Guide to the Brain*, by John J. Ratey, MD, is an excellent introduction to the newer findings of how the brain works, presenting it in a language akin to what the brain uses—analogies and metaphors, and not the computer(binary) approach that is commonly used. Using the theater metaphor—were the entirety of the play will convey a different meaning or feeling than the individual roles could. The interactions of genes, development, anatomical, physiological, environment and life experiences, interact to produce cognitions, emotions and behaviors that cannot be explain by any individual factor. It is a very informative way to look at the same old information.

We also must consider the unique influences of our experiences and cultures. New insights have developed in how culture is superimposed on our genetic code, providing a more flexible and varied fine-tuning of our behaviors. Genetic mutation and natural selection is so slow that we rely on cultural evolution to adjust to our changing environment. That is why culture and socialization is so important for our survival. Unfortunately, due to our incredible diversities, it would take an encyclopedia to explore and explain how cultural and societal pressures influence our behaviors. It is very difficult to generalize unique life experiences. Anyway, you have already learned about these factors from reading the great books. Shakespeare, Cervantes nor Dante needed knowledge in neuropsychiatry to describe the human psyche. Our religious and philosophical writing will address these aspects too. Another reason we need the return of common sense, to sort thru all this information. If society encourages common sense, it will return faster; if not, special interest groups will gain influence and conflicts will increase.

I will like to discuss our new understanding of how the brain works less like a soloist and more like an orchestra. A collection of genes, synaptic connections, structures, neurotransmissions and life experiences memories. Our brain is organized so that when all these players play together, beautiful music is produced. Unfortunately, one player can disrupt the symphony. It does not matter if the disruption is due to trauma to the brain, genetics, or life experiences, the result will be a disjointed performance. We see this in daily life, when a part of us (a player), wants to eat or sleep more, even though we know that in the long run is not healthy. Even if the rest of the players are playing the right tune, that one rebel can affect the whole. These concepts help us understand addiction, where people's actions and behaviors make no sense. One player in our brain's orchestra may want the drug so bad it drowns out the rest of the musicians, even though the whole organism suffers.

This same concept can be applied to other human traits, from how much we eat to our need for love. The addict destroys his life and the lives of those around him. An obese person takes seconds at dinner even when developing Diabetes. Our friend goes back, over and over again, to an abusive relationship. How much common sense is this? It is hard for most of us to understand these behaviors. For one specific craving, be it love, drugs, or hunger, the whole organism suffers. Maybe we see similarities with special interest groups, where advocating for a specific cause is more important than the effects they have on the whole individual or society.

For greater understanding of the "selfish gene" concept, read Richard Dawkins'* *The Selfish Gene.* You may not agree with his conclusions, but it will make you think. A book that is easier to understand and describes concepts we can apply to our daily life is *Mean Genes,* * by Burnham and Phelan. It is an owner's manual to the brain, from an evolutionary biological perspective. They use examples of our daily struggles with love, money, sex, diet, and beauty. They explain that the brain is a constellation of individual genes with their own agendas that, many times, are the basis of our struggles.

A common example is our struggle with weight. In our past, periods of famine were common. Those genes that drove us to pack a few extra pounds on when food was plentiful helped us survive. There was no refrigerator to store food against future need. To survive, they followed a simple rule: eat all the food in front of you; you may not have any tomorrow. Now that we spend our lives behind desks or in front of the TV, with frozen or fast food, and Chinese delivery at our fingertips, that same life saving drive becomes a problem.

This mismatch between the modern world and our genes is at the center of many of our problems. Fortunately, a mind, or individual consciousness, has developed, just like the conductor of an orchestra, who tries to keep all players together for their long term good. We can override these hurtful urges, but it is not easy. As corporate marketing becomes more sophisticated, using and activating our urges or drives like sex, hunger and security, we weaken. Some examples would be super sizing our food for our sugar and fat cravings, scantily dressed models for our sex drives, and TV programs showing extreme behaviors and emotions to satisfy our emotional fantasies. Even our loved ones contribute to our battles, preparing favorite high caloric pies, or buying us a toy we really did not need. That is why knowing how our genes influence us, and avoiding exposure to extreme temptations, cultivating discipline, will make it easier to control these urges. Two thousand years ago, the apostle Paul wrote, in Romans 7:15-17, "I do not understand what I do. For what I want to do, I do not do, but what I hate I do. And if I do what I do not want to do, I agree that the Law is good. As it is, it is no longer I myself who do it, but it is sin living in me." A battle of the flesh or the mean genes— you pick a name.

This is how science, religion, philosophy, morals, or theories of government deal with knowledge acquired through different methods. As science unravels the mystery of our inherited genetic predispositions and the relationship of physical and psychological trauma with hormones and neurotransmitters, are we reducing the roles of other areas of human understanding? As we understand the influences of family, personality, and environment on our motivations, values and choices, will we be able to predict our behaviors?

Could we input this information into a computer and predict what we will do next? Will free will die?

No, "free will" will not die. Many things affect human thought and behavior, and many times we cannot even explain our own actions. As some studies of the disconnect between the right and left hemisphere of the brain have shown, we may never know our original motivation. I will explain this later. Experts have not been able to determine the motivation for behaviors. Concepts like diminished capacity, temporary insanity, and the abuse defense, are a reflection of our arbitrary social and legal defense of certain behaviors.

A person that kills a severely abusive spouse while he is asleep may be excused, because her crime is considered self-defense. If the same woman killed her husband because he hid a key, she would be found guilty, no matter how important her need for the key. Sometimes, when people get intoxicated, they do not remember what they did. Scientifically, it would be easy to prove that an intoxicated person did not remember his actions, knew his motivation, nor possessed the *mens rea* behind his crime. Scientist accepts the concept of blackouts, where the intoxicated person has no memory of what he did. Nevertheless, as a society, we decided that those blackouts would not excuse a person, while in the abuse case, the state of mind was assumed to have rendered the person unable to rationally seek police or court help, even tough it would be more difficult to prove scientifically.

Our society has decided that drunkenness does not excuse someone of a crime. It does not matter that the intoxicated person did not mean to kill a child with his car. There was no *"mens rea"* intent or motivation for killing the child. The drunk could have no memory of his actions, and he will still be found guilty. A democratic society must start with the premise that all individuals are morally, ethically, and personally responsible for their actions—that they possess free will. No matter how strong the urge to drink, the sexual attraction, or the raging anger, one is responsible for one's behaviors. It does not matter if electroencephalograms or functional magnetic resonance imaging shows that the brain lights up when the accused sees a drink, a sexual image, or things that make him angry. If he gives in to his urges, he needs to be accountable.

The message must be clear. If you give in to your impulses, you will pay the price. It is disrespectful to those who do not give in to their impulses to excuse those who do. Being born with a disorder or biological drive, or suffering trauma does not excuse bad behavior. Too often, we think because "we were born that way" it is okay! Most of our laws are to prevent us from disregarding the rights of others and not concerned if the violation was a result of our biological endowment or secondary to trauma because of an accident. It does not matter the way we were raised. If you cannot control your impulses, seek help before the crime, not after. We have many options for help; from spiritual guidance, to different mental health approaches. Many times a combination of these approaches will be indicated.

As a society, we often will not punish someone, when it is found that the individual was incapable of knowing right from wrong; depending on which standard the community uses. They could be found not guilty "by reason of insanity." This is the exception, not the rule. Our laws are a contract with society, and in a way arbitrary. We tend to think that if a crime is biologically based, it is excusable, but it does not matter if a pedophile has a provable genetic, hormonal, or traumatic experience that drives him to seek sex with children, we expect him not to give in, as it is not just about himself but it involves others. He or she should have sought help or curb his drive.

Everyday, we hear of new discoveries that "prove" that developmental, genetic, or traumatic conditions "cause" or "contribute" to undesirable behaviors. Some will pass the test of time, others will not. Does this mean people can give in to their impulses? What about the rights of the victims and their families? While the insanity defense is important for our society, it should be used responsibly. Every time somebody uses this defense, it increases the stigma and shame of those that suffer psychiatric problems and keep them in check. When a headline like, "teacher sexually abuses child because he suffers from a bipolar disorder" appears in the news, my patients who suffer from a Bipolar disorder, tremble. Will their co-workers, neighbors or family avoid leaving them with children now? Will they become pedophiles? No! Their Bipolar disorder when active or untreated may affect their judgment, but will not "make them abuse children." Many times the crime has nothing to do with the problem. Unfortunately, many in the mental health field (acting as a special interest group) will be quoted in the media as blaming the abuse of the child on the Bipolar disorder or the lack of public funds for its treatment. Stigma or prejudice is blamed for preventing the perpetrator from seeking help. In reality, most child sexual abusers do not suffer from Bipolar disorders, and most Bipolar patients will never abuse a child.

Let us explore our brain's subdivisions. See Table II, which summarizes the qualities of the left and right hemispheres of the brain.

Left and Right Hemisphere Preferences	
Left Hemisphere	Right Hemisphere
Rational	Intuitive
Prefers verbal information and instructions	On hand demonstrations
Brakes problems in parts, later connecting in a sequential, logical fashion	Looks for patterns, follow hunches
Is structured and follow plans	Specific instructions not needed
Looks at differences Is a splitter, distinction important	Looks at similarities is a lumper; connect ness important
Controls feelings	Free and loose with feelings
Prefers ranked authority structures	collegial authority structures preferred
Sees cause and effect in a linear fashion ness	Is analogical, sees interconnect
Prefers multiple choice questions	Prefers open ended questions

The right and left Brain hemispheres, process information and emotional content differently. Even though we use both hemispheres for most tasks, we have a dominant side that can overwrite the inputs from the other side. However, acquiring and processing information, and our ability to understand and adjust to our environment, are enhanced when both sides of the brain participate.

The left side of the brain is logical and moves from parts to the whole sequentially. It is good with words and math and follows the rules. The right side of the brain takes a more holistic approach. Rules interfere with the right hemisphere's creativity and randomness; it prefers pictures, sounds, and emotions to words or mathematics. The left side of the brain processes in a linear, sequential, and logical manner, taking the algebraic equation, and solving it section by section until it finds the answer. The right side of the brain uses a more intuitive approach, looks at the whole equation, and solves it without being able to explain how it achieved the solution. Both sides of the brain were probably used, just one more than the other.

The *corpus callosum* is a structure in the brain that connects both hemispheres. Many cases of the deficits and behaviors that resulted when this connection was severed were studied. In the past, a surgery was performed to disconnect the hemispheres, when there were no other treatments for intractable seizures. By separating the connection, they kept the seizure from spreading. This helped us understand the differences between the hemispheres. The left hemisphere controls language and the major motor functions of the right side of the body. Damage to this side could result in the loss of our ability to understand or use language or the move our right arm or leg. The right hemisphere contributes to the emotional coloring of language. There are new findings of the interactions of the right and left hemispheres. We depend on *pattern recognition*—that ability to recognize a new object or situation as similar or belonging to an already familiar class of objects or situations. Otherwise, every object or situation would be a new encounter and we would be unable to use previous experiences to react. Pattern recognition is a powerful mechanism for successful problem solving. The transmission and understanding of information we cannot see or experience is dependent on this. We transmit this information from individual to individual, from generation to generation, via our culture. We do not have to learn everything from scratch. Similarly, we may continue the same errors from generation to generation. We tackle a novel problem with the right hemisphere. We compare it to familiar patterns stored in the left hemisphere. When it becomes a familiar experience, a new pattern can be stored and managed in the left hemisphere.

It is like learning to drive a car. At the beginning, it is very tedious, but as we practice, it becomes automatic. Once we ingrain a pattern in our left hemisphere, it is harder to change. That is why when you learn an activity with the wrong movements or techniques, like a sport grip, it is hard to change. The expression "old habits die hard" has a grain of truth. This could be a contributing factor to why we develop prejudices. David Berreby in his book, *Us and Them*, explores our tribal minds and our tendency to categorize people. It does not matter whether it is ethnic or racial groups, political or religious beliefs, sports teams or neighborhoods gangs—humans kill other humans under the influence of group mentality, the us pattern vs. them pattern.

Another interesting finding is that changes in our brain as we age are related to atrophy of the right hemisphere. This could explain our dependence on pattern recognition as we grow older and it becomes harder to "teach old dog new tricks." Thank God for experiences! However, this is not an absolute. I know people older than me who grasp new concepts faster than I do. Elkhonon Goldberg, PhD, in his book, *The Wisdom Paradox*, explains these concepts and shows us how wisdom grows as we age.

In the 1800s, the railroad worker Phineas Gage damaged parts of his brain, leaving him with emotional and intellectual deficits. This helped doctors understand the localization of brain functions within the hemispheres. Not only are there distinct anatomical areas that control certain functions, there are also interconnecting systems that control or modulate others. Recent studies show that damage to one hemisphere can result in the healthy side running out of control, without the checks and balances of the other side. If a person has a left hemisphere stroke, he is more likely to be pessimistic, even suicidal, whereas if he has a right hemisphere stroke, he will underestimate his deficits and want to leave the hospital early. Even when paralyzed, he may think he could walk. More relevant to our discussion is the finding that if hemispheres are disconnected, how each perceives stimuli may be very different. One hemisphere may not be aware of what the other experiences and the interpretation of events as presented to one side may be very different. For example, if a subject with disconnected hemispheres were presented a written command to pick up a soft drink that only his right eye could see, he would probably do it. The left hemisphere received the command, but not the right hemisphere. If we then ask him thru his left ear, (the right hemisphere will receive this information) why he picked up the soft drink, he may answer, "I was just thirsty."

As the right hemisphere did not receive the command to pick up the soft drink, he tries to find an answer for behavior for which he is unsure of the motivation. This is an extreme example, but it helps us understand how two people observing or evaluating the same facts develop different perceptions of events. There are strengths and weakness to any thinking style, and neural networks will influence the development of common sense.

Over 90% of people are left hemisphere dominant, with resultant right side preference for functions like writing, or throwing a ball. Stanley Coren, in his book *The Left-Hander Syndrome,* addresses differences between right and left-handedness, and the different rates of health problems and accidents in the left-hander. Healthcare professionals, often to the detriment of their patients, do not use this information. Read his research, especially if you are left-handed, as much can be done to reduce accident rates for left-handers. He explores how many characteristics of each hemisphere are intertwined and cannot be separated.

Years ago, many educators encouraged developing and utilizing both hemispheres of the brain. Even in the public schools, the creative and artistic aspects of a child's development, were emphasized, to help develop the right brain. Like every other fad, it has faded away, but some concepts have remained. Certain characteristics are identified by the way one hemisphere processes information. Tests were developed to measure your brain's strengths. For example, people could show percentages of 45% right and 55% left brain preferences or strengths. Developers of these tests think they can measure your preferences or strengths so you can make better career choices, but it has not been scientifically tested.

A simple way to see if someone utilizes more right or left-brain strengths is to ask for directions. If he says, "Go straight for 200 meters, turn right on Main Street, go four blocks, and make a left turn," he is probably a "left-brainer." A "right-brainer" gives these directions: "Go straight until you see the old Wal-mart store and make a right; make a left at the burned building." The left-brainer uses numbers in sequence, whereas the right-brainer uses visual description. Nevertheless, if you and I were lost in a metropolitan area in the middle of rush hour, wouldn't it be easier if someone utilizing both hemispheres gave us directions?

This is the reason artists have a hard time communicating with business people. They have different temperaments, dispositions, strengths, and approaches to life.

Hemispheric strengths are very influential in specialization at work or sports. Even though ten percent of the population is left-handed, in professional golf, none of the leaders is left-handed, (right hemisphere dominant). Even Phil Mickelson, who hits left-handed, is right-handed for activities like writing and throwing balls. So most golfers are left hemisphere dominant as compare to the general population. Contrast that with tennis, where many of its legends were, and are, left-handed and probably R-Hemisphere dominant. Golf is a static, rules-based game of precision. The fans and players are quiet, serious, and control their emotions. Tennis may require more right hemisphere strengths as the ball is constantly moving and every shot will be different. The personalities of the tennis pros show more emotion in and out of the court, than the more serious golfers. Is that why tennis fans are more fun?

We have *pairs* of eyes, ears, arms, and legs. We have twenty-three *pairs* of chromosomes that carry our gene pairs. We have two hemispheres. Could this be why we tend toward binary thinking? Why we prefer two options—black or white, good or bad, conservative or liberal? No, it is not as simple as that.

As you explore nature, this apparently simple, binary thinking, melts into quantum physics, chaos theory, relativity, and the ways our children make decisions. We sometimes wonder about our own decisions; even planning holidays involves many options. Will we fly or drive to visit Cousin Debbie or Cousin Maria, or will we just stay home? Should I leave on Friday or Sunday? So many factors are involved that it is a wonder we even make a decision. Nevertheless, when we make our decision, we usually do not take the time to explain the factors we considered. Other factors we were unaware of considering could have influenced our decision. The right hemisphere lends its power of intuition, which many times cannot be logically explained. If every time we made a decision we tried to explain every reason behind it, we would never finish.

Fast, vivid stimuli—from video games to action movies to thirty-second news clips—are presented as binary propositions. As our lives become more complicated, with less time to do what we must, we depend on the TV news to give us concise information. We depend on the fifteen-second advertisement to educate us. We resort to all-or-none answers because they are easier. We have been conditioned for no or yes, yours or mine, good or bad answer. That is how we first learn our behaviors. As we develop, our choices become more complicated. When presented with many options, we become confused and indecisive. That is why salespeople are trained to give only two options. Do you want the red or the white car? Being aware of our tendency towards binary thinking helps us take information a step further and consider what options were discarded in the fifteen-second presentation. Remember, "they" did the thinking for us and presented their conclusions.

I think it is important to look at our emotions, which unfortunately, can be our worst enemy. Emotions affect our decisions and are more powerful than logic. This is easily understood under the concept of flight or fight. Emotions occur automatically. We cannot plan or choose them. However, we can control what we do with them. Life or death situations require immediate reaction, provided by emotions. Our neo-cortex takes too long. For a comprehensive exploration of emotions and feelings from a scientific point of view, I recommend books by the neuroscientist Antonio Damasio. Binary, dualistic thinking is part of our makeup. It may simplify our lives, but it also can complicate it. Binary thinking is like computer language—on or off, "1" or "0."

Many people believe that everything in our lives, including feelings, emotions, and religion, can be understood with binary thinking, which is why they think a super-computer will create artificial intelligence. I read in the newspaper that a poll of scientists showed that most had selected *Blade Runner* as their favorite science fiction movie. In *Blade Runner*, a corporation develops human-like robots and sets an "expiration date" on them, after which they will self-destruct. A new unauthorized breed of advanced robots is developed. They are so advanced that they figure out on their own, their limited time. They want to live as long as humans and experience emotions. The hero, Harrison Ford, is a cop whose job it is to destroy the renegade robots. The only way to tell the difference between a human and a robot is that the human has memories and emotions associated with them. Were the contacts with humans helping robots developed emotions, which interfere with their original programs? Watch the movie.

Some scientists believe humans will be able to create "artificial humans," but others think it will not be possible. *The Creature*, humans will not be able to figure out the Creator, God or Nature. Other books and movies deal with these themes. The supercomputer Hal, from the movie, *2001: A Space Odyssey*, takes control over the Space Mission. The movie, *I Robot*, based on Isaac Asimov's book, further explores these themes. The robots developed by a corporation to serve and protect humans, evolved on their own. The robots figure out that in order to protect humans, they have to take full control of humans to protect them from destroying themselves. Even tough humans and robots had the same goal of protecting humans they disagreed on the method. While logically it makes sense for the robots to control humans to protect them from themselves, the human are not willing to give up Liberties for security. War erupts and the emotional human triumphs over the logical robot. On the other hand, was it only a logical cost-benefit analysis, were the humans were not willing to give up so much Liberty for their security. Well it sounds like our daily political decisions we make, from taxes to terrorism. It is amazing how many books are written addressing these issues, especially by Nobel Laureates, who vehemently disagree with each other.

At the same time, millions of people think that the answers to these questions were revealed through religion. What is interesting to me is how, even in their selected fields like religion or sociology, experts can not agree. I guess we humans will never completely figure God or Nature out; maybe we can just aim to be *generally right and avoid being precisely wrong. On the other hand, maybe we are just getting it progressively less wrong.*

Summary of Why Johnnie Is a Rebel without a Cause

1. Our birth order and family dynamics affect how we perceive and interact with others.

2. Society plays out the dynamics of families on a large scale.

3. To start understanding societal conflicts, start looking at your own family dynamics.

4. In general, first-borns tend to be leaders. This could explain the high proportion of first-born US presidents.

5. Latter-born tend to be rebels, as earlier children have already taken traditional roles in the family.

6. Middle children tend to be peacemakers between older and younger children, excellent training ground for helping professions and negotiators.

7. Inequality begins at home; in the United States, income inequalities are greater between siblings than between unrelated people.

8. These findings will help you develop your common sense.

Chapter Four

Why Johnnie Is a Rebel without a Cause—Familial Influences

B irth order and family dynamics have a significant influence on how we acquire and process knowledge. Even society enacts the dynamics of a family. If we want to understand social issues, we do not have to go further than our own families. Many studies have been conducted on the influence of the family, explaining why some people rebel or embrace change and others from the same family fight for the status quo. Even though we share fifty percent of our genes with our siblings and parents, and are usually raised in similar socioeconomic environments, studies show that the ways we approach problems are highly diverse. Since Biblical times, we have had sibling rivalry, starting with Cain murdering his younger brother, Abel. Conflicts occurred between our first couple, Adam and Eve. As soon as one got into trouble, the other followed, and the pointing of fingers began.

As a physician, I will address conflicts from a biological perspective. We are born with multiple instincts, including the drive for survival. Examples are: (1) food, (2) reproduction, and (3) personal security. Other drives are also important, like love, certainty, truth, well being, pain avoidance, and spiritual salvation. Some of these drives have influenced us since early childhood, and may cause conflicts within the family. Even though, as parents, we are not very conscious of them, conflicts go on over food, toys, or our attention or favor. From a child's perspective, it is a very real battle for survival. Many societies are blessed with abundance, but in the past, a child's life or death struggle was real. Let us see examples of how birth order influenced the outcomes of conflicts.

The first-born has many advantages; he or she will usually be the most developed and strongest, already having established his or her position in the family. If a crisis arises and limited resources are available, parents may have to choose which child receives them. As the parents have already invested more resources in the eldest child, who will probably be the strongest and have the best chance of survival, most resources will be directed to him/her. This may also explain the custom of primogeniture, in which the eldest son inherits the family's estate, as it would not be economically viable if it were to be divided. In lands where primogeniture rules, the second son might join a religious order, and not marry, which would also prevent the need to divide resources. The third son usually joined the armed forces, possibly creating his own estate. Families also faced similar conflicts with their daughters, depending on their customs and resources. Daughters' roles were similar. Here the options of marriage, caretaking of aging relatives, or joining a religious order, were necessary for survival. This may sound cold and calculating, but this was the common pattern for landed families in Europe. We have come a long way, and usually do not have to make these kinds of decisions. In the United States, with our strong emphasis on individuality, family roles are not destined; still, similar patterns emerge. The first-born son tends to follow the family's lead and is more conservative and less open to change. He is the first child and will always have established first his niche in the family. If his parents are more open to change, the first-born will also be more likely to be open to change. These differences are compounded when gender is considered. In today's society of blended families, interactions and conflicts among stepsiblings multiply and become more complex. We are just starting to find out how these interactions change the dynamics of families, which will affect society's dynamics.

Born to Rebel, by Frank J. Sulloway, includes a comprehensive bibliography and extensive, innovative research that will help you explore these issues. Sulloway tries to understand why some people reject conventional wisdom, and others, equally intelligent, scientific thinkers, defend the status quo zealously. This sometimes results in significant social conflict and even revolutions. Sulloway gives examples of political and social movements, like the French Revolution, in which the supporters of the status quo were often first-born, and the latter-born favored revolutionary changes.

Even first-born that supported revolutionary change tended to be dogmatic and more willing to impose their will. Similarly, to the way they impose their will towards the younger siblings. He could use his strength for the "good of the family," preventing a younger sibling from running into traffic, or to satisfy his selfish wishes—taking away his siblings' toys. Sulloway gives examples of paradigm-shifting discoveries, like Darwin's theory of natural selection. He demonstrated that scientists most likely to fight for the status quo were more likely to be first-born. Those who accepted theory changes more readily were more likely to be latter-born, like Darwin himself. Latter children tend to question traditions, as the first-born already occupied the "traditional family niche." They have to be more resourceful in getting the attention and resources that now are been divided. No wonder the later child is more likely to be a revolutionary.

The middle child must look up to his elder sibling and down on the younger siblings. Because of this, he finds himself in the midst of battles and learns to mediate and keep the peace to avoid getting it from all sides. You can apply these findings to your own family, but also to political and social systems.

I would like to recommend, too, Danton Conley's book, *The Pecking Order*, which takes a different approach to the topic of family and birth order and presents other factors that contribute to success in society. Conley, who describes himself as been liberal, explores the effects of socioeconomics, discrimination, gender, and family size, and cites studies showing that sibling differences represent seventy-five percent of all income inequalities in the US. Inequality begins at home. This is an amazing statement, as it contradicts conventional wisdom, in which race, ethnicity, education, and origin, explain the differences. His studies must be replicated. Conley's book is a good example of how researched knowledge that contradicts conventional wisdom is kept from public intercourse, as it would force many pundits, and their special interest groups, to change their assumptions and beliefs to achieve their goals. It would be hard to acknowledge that what you have been pushing throughout the years as dogma, was wrong. If they used the process of common sense, they would not have to backpedal so much. If the public would see them as special interest groups, then they would not be surprised nor feel taken, as their role was understood, they were just interested in achieving their goal and not how their special pet issue, fitted the general picture of society or the individual.

Summary of "Personality Filters"

1. Personality is a strong filter of how we acquire and interpret information.

2. There are many complex theories of personality, but these four temperament traits— novelty seeking, reward dependence, persistence, and harm-avoidance—will help you understand yourself and others.

3. A simple sentence—"Could you walk the dog?"— could have many meanings, depending on the personality filters of the communicants.

4. The same personality filters also affect the communications of societies.

5. Keep this in mind for your common sense approach.

CHAPTER FIVE

WHY SUZY IS AN ACCOUNTANT AND MARY AN ENTERTAINER

Personality Filters

Many theories have been formulated to explain and assess personality, from the influences of genetics and environment, to questioning whether it is possible to change our personalities. It does not matter whether you take the phenomenological or descriptive approach, use the Myers-Briggs classifications, or adopt in-vogue theories. Common sense will help you understand.

Essentially, I define personality as the set of characteristics that manifest in how we adjust to environmental stimuli—physical, social, psychological, or spiritual. These characteristics are stable, but not permanently fixed. Instead of discussing compulsive or histrionic personalities, we will discuss common sense traits of our personality. Rate your personality and those of the people you know well to understand yourself and others better. You can see a summary of personality traits in Table III.

Personality, Temperament Traits

Dimension	High	Low
Novelty Seeking	Looks for excitement	Avoids new experiences
	Impulsive	Reserved
	Bored easily	Enjoys routines
Reward Dependency	Sociable	Independent
	Sympathetic	Critical
	Warm	Aloof
	Sentimental	Detach, cold
Persistence	Perfectionist	Pragmatist
	Determined, pushes himself	More easily gives up
	Ambitious	Satisfied with status quo
Harm Avoidance	Fearful	Daring
	Shy	Outgoing
	Pessimistic	Optimistic

Others may refer to these traits as "temperament dimensions," but I will avoid confusing you with the different aspects or details. Dr. C. Robert Clonninger's work has helped me understand personality and human development. His book, *Feeling Good: the Science of Wellbeing*, is an incredible synthesis of new biological knowledge with the "classical" approach to understanding the steps people take to achieve contentment and improve self-knowledge. In a scholarly fashion, he integrates biomedical and psychosocial sciences, avoiding a reductionist approach. At times, it may be too technical to the average person, as he includes the science used to prove his points. You may skim thru these parts without missing the main points of his book.

Now, let us explore the personality traits that make us different. Do you cringe at the idea of bungee jumping from a bridge suspended five thousand feet above a river? If so, you rank higher on the scale of *risk avoidance*. If you cannot wait for a new roller coaster ride (or any new experience), then you will rate high in *novelty-seeking* traits. Do you need the approval or company of others and hate to be alone? If you answer "yes" to this question, you are higher on the *reward-dependence* scale. If you prefer to be alone and are an independent thinker, you would be low on that scale. Do you need to follow a daily routine and are not satisfied until your projects are "perfect"? That puts you high on *perseverance*.

As with most things, it is not *all or none*. There are degrees. Take two stereotypical personalities—the accountant and the actor. Go down the list. The accountant will most likely rate high in *persistence*. He is determined to perfect his work on time, following the rules, crossing the T's, and dotting the I's. The actor is more interested in his art, not in time or money. Rules are just a guide, and he crosses the T's only if they look better. In *novelty seeking*, the accountant will probably be low, as he tends to follow rules and not change his habits. The actor's novelty seeking traits will probably be high, as he likes to play different characters. How about *harm avoidance*? Try getting your accountant to take an extra deduction on your tax forms if you do not have the receipts. The actor will invite and test life—from fast convertibles to emotional behavior. While a tax refund may satisfy the accountant, the actor finds reward from the adulation of his fans, as he is likely to be higher in *reward dependence* traits.

I use stereotypes to help people understand these concepts. You can compare other personality classifications with this approach. Someone high in *persistence* and *harm avoidance,* and low in *novelty seeking,* will tend toward an obsessive-compulsive personality. They are often perfectionists, avoid situations where they could get hurt, and prefer familiarity and repetitive tasks.

Relative percentages and interactions of these traits point to personalities once called "histrionic" or "narcissistic" by other theorists. Now, we can see how these traits lead to success in certain professions; even within fields, personality traits can take us down different paths. Can you imagine Britney Spears as the host of *Mr. Rogers' Neighborhood,* or Mr. Rogers dancing and singing at the Grammies? Both found their niche, and both have provided us entertainment according to their personalities.

There is no single, ideal personality for everyone. We each have traits that serve best our roles. Nature and diversity go hand in hand. We need diverse personalities. Traits are not pathological unless they prevent the person from functioning. If your *harm avoidance* is so high that you cannot leave the house, you may need the help of an expert.

How can we apply these concepts to how we acquire and process knowledge? Let us try common sense again. How you perceive the world depends, in part, on your personality. Look at a husband who is rated high in *harm avoidance* and *reward dependence,* while his wife is low in both. The couple has just moved to a new neighborhood, and the wife tells her husband, "You need to take the dog for a walk." What appears to be a simple request is really a conflict-producing statement. The wife does not fear walking in a new neighborhood, so she feels it should not be a problem. The husband grumbles; he feels his wife simply does not want to take the risk, and sends him on the difficult task.

Remember, the wife is low *harm avoidance*, so it does not cross her mind that her spouse may think she is asking too much. He imagines there may be a vicious dog around the corner. He grumbles, feeling that his wife chose the easier task—preparing the meal. He would prefer to cook and not expose himself to the new experience of walking the dog in their neighborhood.

His wife feels that her husband will not even take the dog for a walk because he is lazy. One small request has upset two people. If she understood her husband's personality, she might have reminded him that around the corner, their old friends could be waiting helping him overcome his *fears* by encouraging his reward dependent traits.

The same concept could be applied when discussing national policy changes or fixing a problem at work. If we want to communicate well, we need to speak the same "language", or understand were the other person is coming from. Most of the time, our choice of words, or facts that we chose to emphasize depends on our personality traits of which we are not even aware. Understanding personality traits will help all of us communicate better.

Summary of "The Madness of Crowds"

1. Emotions are stronger than our rational mind.

2. The "herding principle" will help us understand the irrationality that groups sometimes exhibit.

3. The madness of crowds will help explain the phenomena of Beanie Babies, real estate bubbles, and Internet stock speculation. It will also explain political, religious, and social movements that defy rational explanation.

4. Without this understanding, these behaviors make little sense and could interfere with the development of common sense.

Chapter Six

The Madness of Crowds

"I can measure the motions of [celestial] bodies,
but I can't measure human folly."

Isaac Newton

Those words were attributed to Isaac Newton, the obsessive, analytical, mathematical genius, after he lost a fortune in the South Sea bubble. He was caught in the frenzy of stock speculation, and like everyone else, did not take the time to analyze the merits of the investment.

What is it about fads that so many brilliant, prudent people are caught in the frenzy of rising prices and the subsequent crash? Harvey Mackay, in his classic, *Popular Delusions and the Madness of Crowds,** documents other similar episodes in human history. This book can help you gain a perspective of crowd behaviors in different human spheres. Knowing group influences in humans will help you understand many apparently irrational behaviors.

One way to look at the brain is to separate it into three developmental parts. The most primitive part is the brainstem, which controls basic functions like breathing and body temperature. The midbrain is where the limbic system and other important structures lie. This system regulates our emotions, like anger, pleasure, pain, or satisfaction. The herding instinct, which causes species to group together like a herd of horses, also resides in this part of the brain. These areas are driven by instinct.

The latest evolutionary brain structure, the neo-cortex, serves to inhibit our instincts, providing more time for reason, experience, and moral or spiritual awareness to override automatic responses from the midbrain.

This chapter deals mainly with the midbrain, as it is involved in the reactions commonly known as "fight or flight." Imagine a group of zebras feeding by the river. Suddenly, one of the zebras sees a lion sneaking in to attack. The zebra takes off running. The zebra never warns his herd, "Watch out, there's a lion coming", but still, the other zebras start running, too.

This also happens with us when faced with a real or imaginary danger. An automatic instantaneously hormonal and neural reaction occurs. Stress hormones like steroids, and catecholamine neurotransmitters like norepinephrine, are pumped to our bloodstream to get the organism ready to fight or run. The senses become acute, the heart goes into overdrive, pain sensitivity decreases, and emotions become aroused.

The lion is coming! We do not have time to think. Imagine what would happen if we saw a lion coming, and our neo-cortex began analyzing the situation. "The lion is coming at thirty miles per hour. On a good day, I can go twenty-five miles per hour, so it will be a few minutes before he catches me. Are there any trees I can climb? Wait! That lion only looks like a 150-pounder. Maybe I can scare him off."

By this time, you would be lunch! That is why we depend on the midbrain to make us react first and think later. Have you ever wondered why the zebras run and not bunch together and kick the lions away? Imagine two hikers, watching a group of lions getting ready to attack them. One person is sitting on the ground tying his tennis shoes, while the other one frantically screams, "What are you doing? We have to fight the lions! We can't outrun them!" The other person responds, *no, all I have to do is outrun you!*

This story also explains how Internet stock manias end. They think all they have to do is sell faster that the other stockholder. A few people start the trend, and if it catches on, even rational skeptics join in. At the beginning, they resisted the trend. Then some "experts," and even their neighbors, were gloating over their profits. They cannot resist the temptation, everyone is doing it and they do not want to be left behind. Then when the crash happens is like waking up from a nightmare. How could I have done that? I was fooled!

By this time, our rational side takes charge. Then the investigations begin, Congressional hearings are demanded, and a scapegoat is found to explain human folly. New regulations are enacted to try preventing it from happening again. A few go to jail, penalties are paid, and then we feel good, until the next fad takes us into frenzy again. Our memories fade and we repeat past mistakes. Do not get me wrong. Unscrupulous people see what is going on and lie, cheat, and take advantage of us. They should be punished, but let us not place all the blame on them. If we blame others without addressing our own culpability, we will be more likely to repeat the same mistakes.

Different experts blame greed, ignorance, the "lottery mentality," or even sin. We can add our biological underpinnings for the herd instincts. The herding instinct is not a negative trait per se; it could save your life. The problem is that it developed a long time ago, and while it is effective in saving us from lion attacks, it is not very effective for modern life attacks. Our systems sometimes hinder us more than help us. As this system depends on powerful emotions that override logical, rational thinking, we tend to overreact. However, because our technology has advanced so far, we are able to make decisions—instant stock trading, overnight loan approvals, or pulling the trigger of a gun before the rational part of our brain has had a chance to give important input or suggest other ways to deal with the problem.

This is another example of how emotions are more powerful than logic. That is why, when people are losing a logical, rational argument, they bring in emotional arguments. This could also helps us understand, but not approve of, barbarous acts—from following demagogues such as Hitler, to killing innocent people during riots. We must be careful and not participate in activities where our limbic system could cause us to lose our objectivity.

Emotions color everything; unless you are a robot or a computer, you cannot avoid them. We do not need to get rid of them to evolve to a higher level. We need comprehensive understanding of our emotional power, so we can use that power in our decision-making.

Two football quarterbacks manage emotions in different ways and are both successful. They have different ways of managing flight or fight reactions. Quarterback M needs to execute a pass from the pocket, while a few three-hundred-pound players are coming at him. He will have to use denial as his defense mechanism. He will not acknowledge that they are coming to hit him as hard as they can. He needs to concentrate on following the steps he practiced, looking to the right for his first receiver, then to the left if his first receiver is covered. He cannot remember the pain he suffered the last time he was sacked because it will distract him. To the fans, he looks like he has "nerves of steel", (a Joe Montana type).

The second type of quarterback shows emotions and excitement, handling the situation differently. The linebackers are coming to get him, and he feels an adrenalin rush, giving him extra strength and focus. He remembers he did not even feel pain the last time those three-hundred-pounders buried him. He gets "in the zone." He responds to every stimulus in the field, from the grunting or footsteps coming from the left side, to catching a glimpse of the safety coming unopposed in the right flank. This quarterback does not go consciously through all the steps he practiced. He is constantly moving. His decisions are spontaneous, not "by the book," but by the seat of his pants, (Terry Bradshaw type). He is as successful as the other quarterback is.

These two quarterbacks will also show very different personalities off the field—one more reserved than the other will. Which fits you better? Figure out your usual approach to flight or fight stimuli and that of others around you. Coaches that excel in the psychology of players know that rattling and raising the emotional level of the first quarterback may get him off his game (okay maybe not Montana). He knows not to do that to the second quarterback, as that will only raise his level of play. We see this during football season, as players try rattling other players during pre-game interviews. Sometimes, by using this technique with the wrong person, you raise their level of play.

Look at the stands. Have you ever seen "the wave" in action? Try it. It gives you, at least temporarily, a shared experience, a sense of belonging, and of being part of something big. The fans' limbic systems get "in tune with each other," and thousands of individuals melt into one. Nobody has to tell anyone how or when to do it; it is automatic. Just like hundreds of animals running as one, the wave develops. Sporting events, concerts, political rallies, and religious revivals are a safe outlet for our herd impulses, as long as we leave Mr. Obnoxious and Ms. Alcohol and Drugs behind and bring Mr. Civility and Ms. Rational

On the other side of the coin, we are outraged when we see riotous people destroying property and killing people who had nothing to do with their grievances. Often, nonviolent people are caught in these frenzies, committing out-of-character acts. The courts sometimes show leniency for those who commit crimes while under the influence of a crowd, at times with a shorter sentence. For the same reason, the courts have curtailed even cherished rights, like free speech. You can say amazing things in the United States and get away with them, but you cannot yell, "Fire!" in a full auditorium and expect the authorities to respect your free speech rights. Mayhem will ensue, as people run to the exits, many may be run over. The person who entices the crowd is responsible for the acts the crowd commits.

The Lone Ranger, an iconic hero of many western films, also demonstrates how we deal with these impulses. While the townspeople acquiesce to corrupted or powerful men, the hero stands tall. Neither intimidation nor group pressure to comply and not rock the boat; will keep him from doing what is right. How can he withstand the lure and pressure of the crowds? Is it his strong personality, they way he was raised, his spiritual strength, his experiences or perhaps his strength lays in weakness of his limbic impulse? The hero is probably a combination of all of the above. This best represents the individual American hero, the "lone ranger," as seen in many of the characters Clint Eastwood has portrayed, or Batman, who does the right thing in his unique and troubled way. The hero is able to rise above the crowd and the herd impulse and do what is right. He lives life by his own terms. Villains, unfortunately, also live by their own rules. Maybe that is why the anti-hero, or even some of the "bad boys", also has a following.

It is hard to resist our emotions, even though we know the consequences of giving in. We were raised studying Greek and Latin classics, world literature, scientific discoveries, and under the spiritual guidance of our parents or church. From Greek tragedies like *Oedipus Rex*, Shakespeare's *Othello*, or the history of David in the Bible, I was encouraged, like so many readers, to control my emotions. Then, during the nineteen sixties and seventies, while society was cycling into a more "right hemisphere" pattern of behavior, emotions came to the forefront. Icons like Ginsburg or Harvard psychologist Timothy Leary encouraged the exploration and "expansion" of emotions with drugs. Rationality and logic were seen as a "Western Culture" means to subjugate and control its own citizens or even the world. A culture war developed. Mental health gurus began stressing the need to express our emotions, to "self-actualize" and be happy. Other mental health practitioners and their patients were caught in the fire. The social mood was changing, the pendulum swinging. The momentum was increasing; our group consciousness following our herding impulses. Our society was experiencing the pendulum swing from the excesses of the roaring twenties to the sacrifices of the economic depression to World War II. From abundance to economic sacrifice and war. Then the pendulum continued to the less burdensome experience of building up the country and raising families in homogeneous tract housing during the 1950s. During this time of war and rebuilding, individuals had to hold in check their personal needs, as everybody had to sacrifice for country and family.

The pendulum did not stop there; it continued to the other extreme. Generations that had not experienced WWII or the

Depression rejected the lifestyle of their parents, who mainly knew sacrifice of their personal needs for the good and survival of the family and society. Suddenly, the personal needs and emotions of the individual were more important than country, society, or family; the nineteen-sixties were here. Freedom and love trumped sacrifice and long-term planning. As people in the mental health field are attracted to, and deal best with emotions, this was an easy fit, and may have contributed to the perception of mental health fields been antiestablishment. The pendulum then swings back again. These swings are seen in art, like from Classical to Baroque to Neoclassical. In economics, from strong centralize power were the individual rights are restricted for the government opinion of what is good for society, to individual liberties taking more center stages as government power decentralizes.

The conflict between our emotional and rational selves continues. Movies, songs, and soap operas dramatize conflicts between the rational and the emotional. Love and emotions usually triumphs over rational, calculated decisions. Heroes marry for love, not money, the preservationist triumphs over the developers planning to convert an old library into condominiums, and the moviegoers leave the theater happy. The costs vs. the benefits of the library conversion—who would want to see that. The emotion of seeing the little person triumphing over the greedy developer will always be a more compelling story. More people will buy tickets.

Researchers have device studies were groups are form in a very arbitrary way to tests group behaviors. Strangers were divided into blue and red teams, and within minutes, these two groups were exchanging insults and accusing each other of cheating. There were no previous connections in between the participants, the prizes were minimal, and after the event, everybody would go home with no further contact. This shows the power of group mentality, Us vs. Them. Let me also point out many cases of groups accomplishing heroic acts—sport teams, charity groups, or heroes that risk their lives in fires, accidents, or natural disasters. Another example of how some characteristics can be a detriment or a blessing.

A slower spread of behavior can range from the hysteria that spreads through schools and baffles the school and health care officials to alien abduction reports and conspiracy theories. Many of these behaviors spread like infectious diseases. They usually begin in a fringe group, where they may brew for many years before they start to spread. Just like the bubonic plague, or Black Death, which devastated towns and killed millions of people during the Middle Age, crowd behaviors lurk, waiting for the right combination of factors to thrive. Feelings of alienation, hopelessness, and boredom are often all it takes. When there are many discontents, vulnerable people become "infected" with the virus, as they do not have a strong "immune system."

Often, a group or someone chooses a scapegoat for their problems from capitalistic robber barons to Communists; from Jewish bankers or Fundamentalist Christians taking over the world. Then, opportunistic leaders, gifted at activating people's limbic systems, offer to free the people from the enemy causing their problems. Suddenly, the small group develops a sense of belonging and purpose. At the beginning, some see them as another fringe group that will self-destruct. Because they are not taken seriously, the groups thrive and become stronger. As belief gives some people a reason to live and hope to better themselves, they become fanatical. If not stopped early, only drastic measures could stop the spread. We see this pattern in families, neighborhood clubs, or even in issues that affect the country. In a more positive note, the same happens with social or religious movements that benefit all, creating and not destroying, spreading healing instead of destruction.

Maybe this is why zombie and "body snatcher" movies are so popular. The script is always a variation of the same thing: some extraordinary event, like invasion by aliens or rogue businesspersons or scientists conducting illegal experiments, occurs. This event changes people into zombies, which cannot feel love, compassion, or empathy. In turn, the zombies try converting the other humans, destroying them if they cannot. At the beginning of the story, most people do not believe there are zombies, or do not take their threats seriously, so the zombies gain strength. Sometimes a greedy person or organization uses the zombies to gain more power. As the zombies' power grows, humans get tired of fighting and give in to the belief that becoming a zombie will be better after all. A small group of heroes is able to stop the spread of the zombies, and in the end, everyone is convinced of the zombies' false promises and evilness. But unfortunately, not before much destruction. A fresh appreciation and reevaluation of what it means to be human evolves.

Our first reaction is to condemn how we let zombies attacks occur. However, "zombie" attacks may be needed, as we grow complacent with the status quo, forgetting what makes us humans, and how we got there. Some believe that without wars or revolutions, power would concentrate in small groups, who would imposed their ideas and prevent progress. Diversity, which is Nature's way to deal with all kinds of unknown future zombie attacks, like viral epidemics, would be curtailed, and the survival of our specie, Homo sapiens, would be in jeopardy.

Others think that, with continued learning and understanding of human nature, we will not need zombie attacks to change us. We will be able to discuss our differences, have small battles, and change. Maybe that is why we have an adversarial legal system, or why special interest groups have evolved. They are small armies trying to impose their will, which forces the public to adjust or change without major revolutions. Others think the ultimate zombie attack is coming in the form of the Biblical Armageddon. We will not be able to stop it, but the Messiah will return, humans will change their ways, and peace will reign after much destruction. During most conflicts, each party believes they are on the right, or on God's side. Abraham Lincoln best expressed it during the Civil War: "The will of God prevails. In great contests each party claims to act in accordance with the will of God. Both may be, and one must be, wrong. God cannot be for and against the same thing at the same time. In the present civil war it is quite possible that God's purpose is something different from the purpose of either party, and yet the human instrumentalities, working just as they do, are the best adaptation to affect his purpose."

Between the extremes of ideas—emotions vs. rationality, democracy vs. fascism, conservative vs. liberal, God and Nature achieve their purpose, which may be very different from the goals these different groups may have. As history shows, our "human instrumentalities" have frequently involved the spilling of blood and the constant retesting of rehash ideas.

If you want to learn about practical application of the limbic system and the way related structures affect human interactions, read Robert Pretcher, PhD. He views the stock market and its averages as the result of the aggregate interactions of humans making choices with their money.

The tendencies of markets to move from one extreme to the other are just reflections of our herding impulses. He believes we find repetitive fractal patterns in nature that manifest as products of human interaction. Repetitive waves occur, one within the development of a larger one. In the structure of the Nautilus shell, the human ear, the universe, or human evolution, patterns repeat. PI and Fibonacci numbers continue to appear in physics, mathematics, and human interactions. These same concepts can be applied to most human endeavors and not just the stock market.

Dr. Pretcher presents evidence of the repetitive patterns Nelson Elliot described in the stock market and has been able to translate this knowledge to human interactions. His premise, that social moods precede events, is a significant change in our view of human nature. We have tended to associate society's mood (which is an aggregate of the individuals' moods) with the events that preceded it. For example, it is assumed that the economic depression in the nineteen thirties caused the raise of fascism, which led to WWII and the concentration camps. In his model, the reverse is true. The negative mood that developed as part of the human cycle, is what caused the contraction of economic activity and led to the rise of Fascism, the war, and its atrocities. He presents us with a different paradigm—of social moods as the cause and not the effect of cyclical changes. The new science of "Socionomics." You can check his reading in the references, and visit his Web site. Understanding past cycles helps, but the acceptance of any theory will depend on its ability to predict, within an acceptable probability, future events. If his theories stand the passage of time, we will need to adjust our understanding of human nature, using the common sense approach.

Summary of "Name Calling"

1. Neither wishful thinking, abstract theories, nor forced denial will change the fact that a rose is a rose.

2. We have not, do not, and will not, know enough to be certain of our knowledge.

3. For every action there will be a reaction; for every option there will be a trade-off. New solutions will bring new problems.

4. Base your common sense on these principles, even if we are not clear what a rose is.

CHAPTER SEVEN

NAME CALLING

A rose is a rose is a rose is a rose.
Gertrude Stein

I s obesity a disease or willful misconduct? Are we victims of the fast food industry, slaves of our desires, or just plain undisciplined? Are hormones, genetics, lack of exercise, or nutrition to blame for people being fat? From talk show hosts and guests, government officials, and healthcare professionals to representatives of insurance companies, the debate goes on. We cannot even agree that obesity is a disease and insurance should pay for treatment. What is the line between an acceptable weight and obese? Is it twenty-five percent over ideal body weight, or fifty percent? Nobody can tell to a scientific certainty what causes obesity and what might cure it. We know many of the contributing factors, but we cannot identify which are the most important in an individual case. We must depend on common sense until science can answer these questions. The same can be said of other disorders like high blood pressure, diabetes, high cholesterol, obesity and clinical depression. When some of these disorders are together, we call it the Metabolic Syndrome.

My good friend, Victor Davila, MD, a research cardiologist at Washington University in Saint Louis, has pointed out how many similarities he sees between his practice and mine. From changing definitions of what constitutes a disorder, to treatment noncompliance with these life-threatening disorders. We have to recruit family members to try to improve patient compliance with treatments. The risks of not properly treating hypertension, diabetes, or clinical depression are well known, but in some patients, there is a significant degree of denial and hope that they will be able to dodge the consequences. Common excuses for avoiding taking personal responsibility for their treatment: "I am not really sick." "My doctor is just too cautious." "I was just stressed out that day." Sometimes even healthcare providers do not use the research and guidelines for treatment or spend the necessary time helping patients understand the repercussions of their behaviors. The metabolic syndrome is becoming epidemic in today's prosperous societies. Here is another place where common sense can help you jump hurdles.

Hypertension, or high blood pressure, is "the silent killer." It causes significant complications—disability and death. Up to twenty percent of the adult population has high blood pressure, depending on how you define it. Do you require three readings at different times or days? Do you take your reading when sitting or lying down? How long do you wait after you drink coffee, exercise, or get over a stressful situation before measuring your blood pressure? Is 140 over 90 the cut-off reading for everybody, or just young adults? Should consistent readings be obtained before we make the diagnosis? Should treatment include diet and exercise?

Studies to clarify some of these issues and to develop guidelines to help healthcare providers treat patients in the real world are been done. Because of the nature of scientific studies, researchers try to control variables while observing the effects of changing only one of those variables. While this is required for meaningful research, the treating clinician in the real world has to guess how to use this information, as variables that can be controlled in a research environment are a wild card in the lives of most patients. Researchers also have resources usually unavailable in the real world.

Let us complicate things a bit more. Doesn't everybody have high blood pressure at one time or another? Of course, when exercising or after drinking a cup of coffee our BP tends to rise. How do we deal with the ethical questions raised when treating hypertension? If a patient's blood pressure increases after he gains twenty pounds, do we refuse to give him medication until he loses those pounds? Do we "enable" him by giving him medications that lower his blood pressure, allowing him to continue gaining weight, smoking, and not exercising? If we refuse to, we risk the patient having a heart attack because of his refusal or inability to change his habits. Should we pay, thru insurance premiums, for the patient's refusal to change his habits? However, how much of the hypertension is related to genetics, the way he was raised, or culture? Is it his fault? Science may not be able to give a certain answer; we will need to use common sense.

These are questions that healthcare professionals and the public wrestle with everyday, most of them arriving at different conclusions. I have practiced in academic centers, mental health centers, and private practice, from large cities to small towns. How communities answered these questions, differed significantly. Standards of practice, treatment of certain diseases, and responsibility differed in many respects. Some communities did not view obesity as a disease, but a personal choice. While some blamed the individual for his obesity, others blamed society, family, ignorance, hormones, fast food, or marketing. What insurances would cover, and physicians would treat reflected the community's beliefs.

The advent of the Internet, with its instant information and available different points of view, paradoxically, contributed to a uniform standard of practice. The development of practice guidelines and evidence-based medicine made a significant contribution to medical practice. This is not to imply that every situation should be uniform, but to stress how improved communication between providers and patients has contributed to more effective treatment plans.. Let us now see how we can apply common sense in the field of psychiatry.

Protect me from my friends; I can protect myself from my enemies.

This common saying describes how many of us in the mental health professions feel. It is also the feeling of many patients, their families, and other health providers.

The more than 250 mental health schools have frequently led battles against themselves with dogmatic, not scientific, approaches. The attacks have often been fratricidal and the name-calling and accusations have grown worse. Social camps believe that psychiatric symptoms should not be diagnosed or labeled because they are related to social injustice. Legal and political conspiracy camps believe diagnosis is a method of social or political control and say patients should be liberated from the shackles of the system. Some push to understand ethical and spiritual dilemmas as a matter of cause and effect, a twisted molecule here or there. The authoritarian camps battle over every word and spin those words to fit new scientific discoveries. How many patients, or their families, resign themselves to hallucinations and depression because of the psychiatric theory in vogue at the time?

Thomas Szasz, MD, the popular psychiatrist, frequently wrote about the myth of psychiatric disorders— that they were not based on scientific principles and were just society's way of controlling dissenting, or "different," individuals. With the explosion of scientific research during the latter part of the 20th century, in epidemiology, neuropharmacology, and neuro-radiology, I wonder if Dr. Szasz has changed his views. With new technology showing significant differences in structure and physiology between schizophrenic and not schizophrenic patients, has he retracted some of his beliefs? I would not be surprised to learn that he has not. Even in the 1950s, he could have discussed his ideas with other doctors, like Robbins and Guze of Washington University or Sir Martin Roth, MD, from England. They had innovative methods of understanding human behaviors and did not narrowly apply the deductive approach Szasz did to knowledge. Szasz did not understand the epidemiological methods that have served us so well. He defined diseases by pathology and laboratory findings, not through the epidemiological or phenomenological approaches used with psychiatric disorders, hypertension, or diabetes. His ideas influenced many people, especially in the legal fields, as he mainly used the deductive/inductive approach to these questions. The problem was that the starting premises were wrong and what followed was flawed. Even some modern celebrities use their notoriety to push an agenda without confirming their information. Reading Dr. Szasz's work, it appears he had good intentions, but approached the issues of psychosis from a legal perspective, elaborating his statements with his gift of applying argumentative deductive reasoning. Dr. Szasz's writings probably helped protect the rights of patients with psychiatric disorders, keeping them from being railroaded into state hospitals and custodial care, as very few effective treatments existed then. It forced society to deal with devastating illnesses that prevented citizens from exercising their rights and duties and made it difficult to look the other way.

However, if we followed Szasz's definitions of illness or disorder, certain serious ailments like epilepsy or migraine headaches would not be identified and treated. Years ago, millions of people with diabetes would have gone undiagnosed, under Dr. Szasz's rubric, as we did not have the technology to measure the sugar or glucose levels in our systems. Diabetes, and the need to treat it, was present before we had this technology. Originally, physicians observed symptoms and complications of diabetes, like kidney failure or blindness. Researchers developed theories even though they did not understand the pathology. As knowledge advanced, theories were discarded, and others were developed. It would have been an incredible disservice to humanity if a hundred years ago we had refused to treat diabetes as a disease. Treatments of this deadly disorder would not have advanced.

We are familiar with the "fasting blood glucose," which measures our glucose levels after fasting overnight. We try to keep our glucose numbers under 100, as complications result from higher blood sugars. When we eat, our blood glucose (sugar) goes up (usually over 100). Insulin and other hormones are secreted in response to this peak, and your organism regulates the glucose back to the levels experienced prior to eating. Having a high glucose reading does not make you a diabetic. Everybody's sugar goes up after eating. The National Diabetes Data Group has redefined a "normal fasting blood sugar" over the years. Years ago, you had to have a fasting blood glucose level over 140 mg/dl. Later studies showed complications at these levels, so to qualify as diabetic you only needed a fasting blood glucose reading higher than 126 mg/dl. Just recently, it was changed to anything over 100 mg/dl. This is a good example of how a disorder is redefined as we learn more about it. We try *getting it progressively less wrong*. It is a work in progress, not set in stone. After we lowered the threshold for who had diabetes, thousands of people were labeled as ill. It had advantages and disadvantages. It helped them get needed treatment, but also make it harder to obtain health insurance. It meant a change in lifestyle, diet, and exercise, and they were suddenly labeled as been different. Society, insurance companies, and even coworkers will treat him differently. His insurance premiums went up, and nobody offered him cake at the office party. Everywhere he would go the Label would follow him.

Why we do not hear complaints of been labeled with a new disease? Why don't we see activists marching down the streets, protesting the conspiracy of healthcare professionals to control human behaviors? Where are the allegations of how the pharmaceutical companies plotted to create and change the definition of diabetes to fool the public and healthcare professionals into adopting "better" medications? Nowhere, as we can understand that identifying a person with diabetes outweighs the possible problems. Let us review again diabetes history.

Diabetes was originally identified by a constellation of symptoms, which usually were the resultant complications patients developed after years of living with high glucose. There was no way to measure blood sugar years ago. Some symptoms were increased thirst and urination, and dizziness. All of these symptoms had to present together, as many other things could cause a sufferer to be thirsty or dizzy. The importance of making a correct diagnosis, even without been able to measure the blood sugar, could be life saving. In the beginning, doctors or researchers caught and treated obvious cases, those with sugar levels in the 300s, testing victim's urine, and monitoring complications, such as dehydration. As our technology improved, laboratory tests were developed to measure blood sugar, connecting blood glucose levels and symptoms and complications. These help connect better the levels of glucose and the symptoms or complications and better treatments evolved.

Let us review. First, doctors recognized diabetes by signs and symptoms commonly found together. As they collected more information and made observations while treating their patients, they were able to categorize different types of diabetes and different etiologies or contributing factors. This aided communication between physicians and avoided errors in research. We learned to treat different types of diabetes differently—pancreatic failure diabetes is not handled the same as diabetes caused by obesity. Now we know that the most common cause of diabetes is insulin resistance, not just "having too much sugar." What was once the cause has become the effect.

Let us go thru a hypothetical case to illustrate how to use common sense to avoid special interest groups taking us down the wrong road. What would happen if nutritionists started assuring us that diabetes was caused by consuming too much sugar and the only effective treatment was diet? If this had happened before we understood the different types and causes of diabetes, progress would have halted. Everyone with diabetes would be prescribed a low-sugar diet, and those whose sugar did not drop would be accused of cheating on their diets. When a scientist published a paper highlighting cellular insulin resistance, special interest groups would attack him. As many businesses and treatment programs would have been developed to provide low-sugar diets, research findings that contradicted this approach would be attacked by all areas of society, not just nutritionists. Progress would be halted. That is why we need common sense to keeps us from becoming entrenched in ideas. Who knows how our Diabetes knowledge will change twenty years from now. When special interest groups become vocal and push their agenda, much useful research is deterred. This scenario never occurred in diabetes research, but in psychiatry, it occurs too frequently. I do not hear "pundits" in the media blasting the pharmaceutical companies for meeting behind close doors and suddenly overnight, declaring millions of people as suffering from diabetes, while planning to sell them new expensive medications. Obviously, I am been sarcastic and this has not occurred with Diabetes, but I hear these complaints all the time regarding psychiatric disorders.

Science is a work in progress, and scientists disagree about where to draw the line. How do we address the need for treatment? We do not want to force diet and/or exercise on all, so we add medications, like Glucophage. Sometimes insulin, via a painful injection, must be administered twice a day. This could cause an infection, or even result in a hospitalization, if he gets his dosage wrong. Fortunately, insulin pumps are now available, so injections soon will be outdated.

Where are the protests of this "barbaric" treatment? Why are these daily injections accepted, but effective, rarely used procedures in psychiatry, like medications or electro-convulsive therapy blasted as barbaric? Both works, but people are more willing to accept the daily insulin injections and even surgery were their body is mutilated, than even taking an effective psychiatric treatment. Even talking about taking medication for affective disorders causes such a ruckus. I am sure that many modern surgeries will be viewed as barbaric in the future, but for now, they can save lives, and we accept them. The ghost in the machine and dual essence conception of body and mind lingers on, and prevents many from receiving effective treatments.

Many studies prove the effectiveness and safety of electroconvulsive therapy (derisively called "shock treatment"), if the diagnosis and the right patients are selected appropriately. Special interest groups have called for its ban, even though it has helped and will help many. It is done mainly on a voluntary basis with the patient's family and significant others consenting to the treatment. Many safety procedures are in place, including requiring a second opinion by another psychiatrist, medical clearance, and having an anesthesiologist present during the treatment. That is more stringent than many surgeries, but people accept surgeries with a lower rate of improvement and greater complications because they believe the illnesses surgery treats are real, while psychiatric problems are caused by stress, society, pharmaceutical companies' profit motives, or psychiatrists that represent society's need to change anti-establishment behaviors. I do not blame the public for this belief, as I have explained before the profession is also to blame.

Mental health professionals have been lax, unscientific, and have not used common sense in defining and differentiating disorders from the depression or anxiety that we all experience. The same way that having high sugar does not make one a diabetic, being depressed, does not qualify one as having a depression disorder. A trick question I ask healthcare professionals during my talks is, "Can you diagnose a patient with 'major depression' if he is not depressed?" The answer is yes. The most used diagnostic criteria for psychiatric disorders are in the DSM-IV. Major depression does not require the symptom of depression if there is an inability to enjoy pleasurable activities. Why we are still calling it "major depression"? Many reasons are given, from tradition, to the historical beliefs that there is no qualitative difference between the feeling of depression and the disorder of depression—just degrees of severity. No wonder the public is confused; the experts cannot agree.

Do an Internet search on *psychiatry* or *mental health*, or go to a bookstore and read some of the titles available in the self-help section. You will find books like *Toxic Psychiatry,** and *Warning: Psychiatry Can Be Hazardous to Your Mental Health.** Many of them written by psychiatrists! The internet search will reveal large organizations that "expose the dangers and evil of psychiatry." Organizations comprised of ex-patients and mental health practitioners have created web sites attacking psychiatry from all angles, accusing psychiatry of "selling out" to the neuroscientists, reductionist philosophers, or "Big Pharma." These same professionals accuse all of psychiatry of trying to usurp religion and spirituality. You will find nearly any opinion—not just from fringe groups, but also from professionals.

I believe in open discussion and considering all points of view, but discussion has to be carried out in an atmosphere of civility. Are we talking about philosophical, scientific, religious, or legal viewpoints? Can we acknowledge that we do not know enough, or could be wrong? Without our friend Ms. Civility, discussions degenerate into a mud fight. That is why I recommend reading *Civility*, by Steven L. Carter. He can reacquaint us with this long gone friend.

I wish these organizations would stop attacking psychiatry, as if it were a monolithic monster ready to devour the world. Psychiatry is just a name used for a field of study. It does not represent a way of life. Those who practice or study psychiatry may have a particular view of what their field represents and may even see it as "the way." Debate their point of view, but do not act as if all practitioners are part of their worldview, nor of a conspiracy to usurp your believes.

Everyone, at one point or another, suffers psychiatric symptoms, like depression or anxiety, contributing to the confusion about what constitutes a disorder in need of treatment. Who has never felt depressed? Is not depression a natural, universal emotion that expresses disappointments or loss? Is not depression part of the healing process when we lose a love one? Most people will answer yes to these questions. It is like pain or anger—a way for our system to tell us something is wrong. The problem arises when the word "depression" is used with different meanings. When the public says, "he is depressed," it most likely refers to a temporary emotion. When mental health professionals refer to depression, they are describing a constellation of signs and symptoms, including insomnia, anxiety, poor concentration, and suicidal ideation. A physician or psychiatrist may use the term to describe a syndrome, or a specific disorder with particular etiology and treatment. So depression could be used to describe a routine emotion, ("my friend is moving out of town and I feel depress"); a more prolong emotional reaction (grief), a syndrome, (depression caused by drugs like steroids), or a specific disorder related to the deregulation of neurotransmitters, like serotonin or norepinephrine. The first two will not need treatment, the syndrome caused by steroids can be repaired, by stopping the steroids, and the specific disorder can be treated with an antidepressant and psychotherapy. Why can't we name all this episodes differently and not just depression? Simply, special interest groups will fight it to the end.

That is how people get confused. Is depression a emotion, a symptom, a syndrome, or an illness? It could be one or all of the above. Major depression is defined in the DSM-IV-R as a constellation of signs and symptoms after other disorders are excluded. It emphasizes the natural history of depression and gives other descriptive findings. This is a huge step forward. I wish they had used a less confusing name, one that could not be misinterpreted or misused. People use the word "depression" to describe an emotion, which makes it harder to understand the concept of a disease in which the *emotion of depression* is just one of the findings of the disease. At Washington University, to avoid some of this confusion, the disorder of depression was called an *Affective Disorder*. Research using the Robbins and Guze concept of how to define a disorder in a patient's presentation, was used to arrive at the Feighner criteria, which later served as a model for the break-through *American Psychiatric Association Diagnostic and Statistical Manual of Mental Disorders* (DSM-III). I think the DSM-IV has continued this tradition of describing symptoms and signs that go together in clinical presentations; I wish they had used different names to describe the disorders to avoid so much confusion.

It is remarkable that the DSM has survived the passage of time, political pressure, and special interest groups. I find it too broad, but I can live with the compromise. For a better explanation and a more complete exploration of disorders, diagnoses, phenomenology, research, and related issues, read Dr. Guze's books and articles in the bibliography.

Depression, just like diabetic patients, gives healthcare providers a constellation of symptoms and signs, including lack of energy, which is found more commonly than feeling sad, insomnia, and crying spells. The healthcare provider tries to figure out what causes these complaints. He completes a history, performs a physical exam, and checks the patient's mental status. He then decides which blood tests or studies are necessary to confirm or rule out other possible causes of the patient's depression, then he develops a diagnosis and treatment plan. There is an important caveat we need to follow. Not only can medical and neurological disorders present with psychiatric symptoms, but also social, developmental, or spiritual factors may contribute to or cause some of the symptoms. A good evaluation should include assessment of these factors, and if appropriate, a referral to a minister, therapist, or any other individual the evaluator deemed necessary to meet the needs of the patient.

The diabetic person might also need a referral. After the healthcare professional completes his evaluation, he may conclude that it is diabetes caused by weight gain and a poor diet. He could refer the patient to a nutritionist and an exercise program, if inactivity was a significant factor or a counselor if the weight was due to stress-triggered eating. The point here is that we can make similar arguments for diabetes and affective disorders.

Just as we have found different types and causes of diabetes, we have also found different types and causes of depressive disorders, from bipolar disorder to dysthymia. Medications used for hypertension or steroids are well known to precipitate depressions indistinguishable from the primary affective disorders. Hormonal imbalances are also implicated. You need an experienced clinician who can help discern the correlating factors affecting your depression.

Is everybody with "depression" in need of treatment or medication? This is a frequent criticism, presented as a question. We also could ask if everyone with high blood sugar or high blood pressure needs treatment or medications. Earlier, I presented times where the blood pressure or blood sugar could be high and not represent a pathological state, just a temporary change in homeostasis. The same way we do not treat these cases, we would not treat depression or grief unless there were other symptoms.

If you have depressive syndrome or disease, should you be treated? Each individual could choose from the different treatments available or none at all. The same way a mild-moderate diabetic could choose from diet, exercise, medications, or insulin, the person with depression has choices—changing life styles, diet, exercise, counseling, psychotherapy, faith, self help, family or group therapy, medications, ECT (electroconvulsive therapy), or new technology, like VNS—vagal nerve stimulation. Obviously, it would depend on the causes, the contributing factors, and the severity of the depression. Some of these options may not be appropriate in certain cases. The professionals are trained to present to the patient the different diagnostic and treatment possibilities, revealing the risks and benefits of each treatment. I usually recommend the presence of a loved one, as severe depression can affect a patient's ability to process information and make a decision. Studies show that if depression is not treated, the risk of alcoholism, obesity, and heart disease increases significantly. Even work productivity diminishes. Surgeries have a higher rate of failures if the patient is clinically depressed.

Okay, get upset, "Mr. Insurance." Let us hear arguments that if insurance companies were required to pay at the same rate for treatment of clinical depression and other psychiatric disorders, it would bankrupt the country. Did diabetes or high blood pressure treatment bankrupt the country? No. We are healthier as a nation. We do not have to pay for treatment for the heart attacks and strokes we would suffer if diabetes or high blood pressure were not treated. The same "savings" would happen with treatment of the disorder of depression, as it would lower the risks of developing or exacerbating other medical disorders.

You have heard the epidemiological large population studies, like the Epidemiological Catchments Area,* that show that approximately twenty to thirty percent of Americans have a psychiatric syndrome during a course of a year. Or that over two thirds of the population will have a psychiatric disorder during their lifetime This statistics are frequently misused to advance some special interest agenda. We do not know if a population that screens positive for the questions asked would qualify for the disorders if they were evaluated in the healthcare provider's office. In addition, a "syndrome" like phobia to a snake could add that person to the study's positive findings. If we identify and exclude similar problems, the percentage of affected individuals would decrease. As we humans have a finite response (behaviors or emotions) to stimuli, some of the screened syndromes identified in the population may represent normal adjustments of our systems, trying to maintain homeostasis, and are neither pathological nor in need of treatment. They are just going through an adjustment period for a specific situation. A good example would be "grief," which all of us go through with the loss of a loved one. Most symptoms of major depression would be present. We know it is temporary and will take its course, sometimes with the help of our families or ministers. However, it will not require psychiatric treatment or medications. The screening test could identify this, and similar situations, as a "psychiatric case." That is the nature of screening tests. They cannot make a diagnosis—only identify who could possibly have a disorder.

Sometimes, either requiring another symptom or eliminating one could give different results, with the percentage of people identified as having a disorder drastically changed.* Ongoing studies are trying to better define who is in need of treatment. This is why people selected at random, taking a non-validated, popular screening test, may appear to have many disorders. A more in-depth evaluation is needed to make a diagnosis. Two people may check the column for anxiety in their screening test. However, there is a significant difference between the person anxiously waiting his cancer test results and the person suffering paralyzing anxiety and panic attacks for no apparent reason. As we adjust for all these factors, you can see that the system will not be overwhelmed. In fact, not getting treatment for serious disorders is a more common problem.

A few years from now, disorders may require different criteria than we have currently. Researchers already predict that psychiatric diagnoses will be classified by neuronal system or neurotransmitter dysfunctions, not by their symptoms or behavioral manifestations. Instead of Major Depression, it could be Amygdale or serotonin dysfunction. That does not mean we do not know what are we doing now, as we have studies and experience, showing that when a certain history and symptoms are present, patients will respond to certain treatments.

Some special interest groups would like you to believe that healthcare providers are just agents of society, trying to control ignorant victims. Even though many of the treatments used in the past have been found marginally effective and discarded, others have been improved upon, getting it progressively less wrong. We all are better off. By conducting double-blind control studies, we should be able to chose more effective treatments or identify who would benefit most from what type of treatment. With the advent of genetic sciences, we will be able, in the near future, to individualize treatment, choosing medication more effective for a particular case and avoiding adverse events.

I will like to address another important point that many times is not considered in our discussions. Most psychiatric disorders are episodic as the patient returns to his previous level of function or at least Improves significantly. This is an important concept, as most people think that once you are "labeled" or diagnosed with a "mental illness" or "psychiatric disorder," you will suffer from it for the rest of your life. An example is major depression, which if untreated, will last around one year. A percentage of depressed patients may become a "chronic case" and will need long-term treatment. Typically, patients with chronic disorders are identified as mentally ill. Nevertheless, most who go through depression manage to function well in society. Abraham Lincoln, Theodore Roosevelt, Prime Minister Winston Churchill, and other well-known celebrities were depressed. These people remained out of the public eye during their acute episodes of depression, but they returned to their previous level of function and were able to contribute significantly to our well-being. Some historians believe that these episodes of depression helped these heroes obtain a level of insight into human suffering, and ultimately gain strength of character, that their accomplishments would not have been possible without these experiences. Unfortunately, this is not the case for many who suffer from these disorders. Even more severe cases like Schizophrenia have been known to remit completely or improve significantly. (A popular example was presented in the movie *A Beautiful Mind,* which explored the life of John Nash, the brilliant mathematician struggling with psychosis).

People should use common sense. Given available information, they can make informed decisions and decide which treatment to try. No matter which treatment they choose, (including no treatment at all), tradeoffs and consequences will happen. For those whose psychiatric disorder is severe enough that it interferes with their ability to understand their choices, loved ones, sometimes with the help of the courts, act as the safety nets. There will be significant unmet needs, especially in the most severe cases, as the social and economic consequences of these disorders are a more difficult challenge. We do not need a one-size fits all approach.

Special interest groups, that forget or do not consider, how their particular interest fits in the whole picture, contributes to the stigma patients and their families suffer. Members of the mental health professions acting as special interest groups, contribute to this stigma. Calling the public or their representatives, ignorant, heartless, or cheap because they do not implement their agenda is misguided. Most people are very generous, volunteering time and contributing money to many causes they understand. As the different special interest groups within the mental health field battle in public over their own dogmatic view of mental health issues, the public becomes more confused and unable to discern between these conflicting information. They expect the public to forget what they learned from their families, religious institutions, philosophical and political spheres, of how the brain, mind, spirit, and society work. Experts with their PhDs. and M.D.'s in the same field, mental health, have such a completely different sets of beliefs about what causes behavioral and emotional problems and ways to treat them, that it is easily understood why the public walks away and does not contribute with their time or money. The public does not have to deal with these fights between the professionals and advocates of cancer or heart disease! It is also easier to understand the issues related to cancer and heart disease as there is greater consensus of contributing factors to these disorders. We have the technology to see the cancer or measure blood pressure so there is less conflicts.

While diabetes or cancer have been recognized as specific diseases in the twentieth century, most psychiatric disorders have been described via observation of behaviors for thousands of year. Explanations have ranged from "black bile" dysfunctions during Aristotle's time, to devil possessions in the Middle Ages. In the last decade, organizations have promoted theories ranging from unconscious, unresolved drives, to social forces or chemical imbalances for the same presenting problems. You do not need to be a rocket scientist to realize something is very wrong! We in the mental health fields should stop pointing fingers until we become more organized. The process of common sense will be a good start.

Do you really expect the public to reach a working consensus when professionals cannot? Do you expect them to open up their wallets for causes they do not understand, or that appear to go against their social, religious or political beliefs? Until professionals can reach a better consensus and be more open about our profession been a work in progress, they will not. We, in our profession, need to better define terms and keep our areas of expertise in very specific problems, avoiding the all encompassing claims of been experts in fields like religion, philosophy, medicine, etc. Maybe evidence-based medicine or disease management programs will help the public understand that treatment and research can be disseminated through a common sense approach. The writings of Dr. Guze have already set the foundation, all that is needed is to restudy them and adjust to well research findings. Perhaps then, the public and other health care professionals will be more willing to seek treatment and open their wallets to support these causes.

The time for calling these disorders "mental illness" has passed. It is time we call them for what they are: Schizophrenia, Bipolar, or Panic Disorders. Lumping heterogeneous disorders into the rubric of mental illness only adds to the confusion and prevents people who need help from getting it. The public can avoid confusion by calling each problem what it is, just as they make a distinction in between hypertension and angina. When referring to general disorders, we could use neuro-psychiatric disorders, a more appropriate designation. Maybe the concept of mental illness should be reserved for the legal sphere, identifying only those patients whose disorder interferes with their ability to form criminal intent or know right from wrong. Procedures for assessing competency to enter into contracts will have to be approached on an individual basis, as there are different standards by which to measure competency. A person who suffers from schizophrenia may be as competent, to vote or form criminal intent, as somebody who does not have the disease. I have also seen a person without a diagnosable neuro-psychiatric illness plead innocence in court because of temporary insanity. The days of the Durham rules, where having a mental disorder automatically meant diminished responsibility or acquittal, are gone. Neither separating the "worried well" from the severely mentally ill patients will not help, as some psychiatric advocates propose. This will contribute to the stigmatization, separation of patients from the mainstream, and increase the public's fear of the mentally ill.

Many organizations call for more government funding for the treatment of "mental illness" in special mental health centers or programs. Usually they are not in the same physical area and do not belong to a general medical system. How is this much different from "send them up-river to the state psychiatric hospital"? Years ago, healthcare professionals in metropolitan areas, would send people who exhibited or reported psychiatric behaviors for treatment at state psychiatric hospitals. The state hospital, due to lack of resources, many times served as custodial facilities—no treatment or rehabilitation was available. They were located far from patients' homes, and as a result, neither family nor friends could visit or monitor treatment. Once a patient was admitted, it was hard to be discharged; the average stay in the hospital was over a year, and some patients spent the rest of their lives there. Many movies and books present the issues patients encountered from a sociopolitical point of view, like *One Flew over the Cuckoo's Nest*; anyone who read the book or watched the movie grew steadfast against seeking psychiatric treatment, which was mainly state or federally funded, putting it at the mercy of the politicians. Patients and their families were too embarrassed to advocate for their needs. If you or your love one were sent for treatment, it felt like you were going to prison. Communication with the outside world was minimized. Families and friends were often prohibited from visiting or communicating with patients. Many reasons were given—from needing to isolate the patient and reduce his stress to accusing the family of being the cause of their disorder.

What would you not do to avoid being identified as mentally ill? You would probably tolerate voices, paranoia, and depression to avoid been sent to one of those psychiatric hospitals. More recently, you could be sent to a mental health center closer to your home, but still it would be isolated from mainstream healthcare. Under the umbrella of confidentiality, your family would find it hard to gain information about you, as these facilities would not even acknowledge that you were there. During the last part of the twentieth century a movement towards private hospitals and services developed. Better facilities and specialized treatment evolved. Advertising by these entities and more recently by pharmaceutical companies, brought mental health issues out of the closet into the mainstream. Unfortunately, many forces, including themselves, contribute to their demise with the pendulum swinging backwards again. Mangled (manage) care taking over. The mystery, isolation, and confusion surrounding the treatment of these disorders continue. The group identification of mentally ill contributes to the "us against them" mentality that I already addressed, and their separation from the mainstream.

It surprises me that bright and dedicated people fight so hard to keep the walls up. They fight for extra funding for a separate National Institute of Mental Health, for separate mental health centers, and special programs. Some professionals tried highlighting cases where violence was committed by patients with mental illness, so the public would demand more programs and involuntary commitment for treatment of the mentally ill. This contributes to stigma, prejudice, and viewing and treating patients as different, in need for isolation for the protection of all. Then the yes, they need treatment, "but not in my backyard" mentality will follow. Highlighting the fact that Charles Manson, the serial killer, could have suffered from paranoid schizophrenia is an insult to the ninety-nine percent of schizophrenic patients, who even in the depths of their psychotic breakdowns would not commit murder.

When President Reagan, Mr. Common Sense himself, uttered the famous words, "Mr. Gorbachev, tear down this wall,"* he was challenging the representative of the Communist government to let people of East and West Berlin mingle to exchange ideas, understand each other's points of view, and make their own choices. The government, President Reagan represented, did not need to build walls or prevent its citizens from communicating with others, so he was not afraid for the wall to come down. We need to get people with serious psychiatric problems back into the mainstream, not away from it. We must destroy walls, not build new ones in the name of confidentiality, compassion, or specialty programs.

Policies instituted decades ago, when we had less knowledge and fewer treatments available, are now obsolete. State hospitals, mental health centers, and other institutions created to relieve families are keeping families apart. Even the original purpose of mental health centers—bringing treatment closer to home—fails us. We must tear down another wall. It is not that these systems are not providing needed services, but with a better understanding of psychiatric disorders and treatments, we will not need to separate or isolate people with psychiatric problems. This also implies hard work for the patients. If they do not keep up with treatment and meet their societal obligations, they will face discrimination. If they want to be treated as equal, they should expect the same responsibilities. For every action, there is a reaction. For every policy change, there is a tradeoff. New solutions will create new problems. Let us apply what has worked in other fields and not isolate ourselves.

Mr. President, Mr. Public, Mr. Healthcare, and Mr. Patient: *Tear down these walls!*

Summary of "Prozac Nation"

1. Life is so complex and changes so rapidly that no human-conceived system, no matter how scientifically based, can explain and predict life.

2. There is no free lunch.

3. Every choice has trade-offs.

4. The challenge is to be generally right and avoid being precisely wrong.

5. Aim to get it progressively less wrong.

6. Knowledge is about the past, thinking is about the future. This is just common sense.

Chapter Eight

Prozac Nation

The challenge is to be broadly right
and avoid being precisely wrong.

O ne group of medications causes approximately 16,000 deaths each year in the United States. Millions of people have used these medications for decades. Their side effects have lead to much suffering and can be worse than the disorder for which they were taken. They are one of the major causes of death by overdose, and more than five hundred children under the age of six die from them each year. Fatal allergic reactions, and more recently, "withdrawal" syndromes are described for people taking them for more than three months.

No, I am not talking about antidepressants. I mean good old aspirin and non-steroidal anti-inflammatory drugs (NSAIDS), like Ibuprofen and Naproxen. You can buy them over the counter. It would be hard to find many houses in America without these medications. They are an effective treatment for pain, inflammation, and fever. Nevertheless, with so many deaths and adverse effects, why do we not see media reports, class action suits, FDA black boxes, and recalls? Because they help, they are generics and there are no big pockets to go after.

In the news more recently, the Cox-2 inhibitors, like Vioxx and Celebrex, gained widespread use for indications of NSAIDS, because they did not have side effects like ulceration or bleeding, as seen with aspirin and NSAIDS. Physicians switched many patients to these drugs, concerned with the side effects of the older drugs. Patients appeared to improve without adverse effects, physicians were happy with their patient's improvements, and pharmaceutical companies' profits soared. It looked like a win-win situation, except for the cost to health insurance companies, who had to pay much more for the new medications. Direct-to-consumer advertisement, like television ads of happy senior citizens dancing, expanded the use of these Cox-2 inhibitors. After approval, research continued, and a possible increased risk of heart attacks and strokes in users, was uncovered. Did companies withhold this information, or did their scientists require more proof before accepting the higher risk of heart attacks? The FDA did not pull the products from the pharmacies, nor did they demand the "black box warning." Merck pulled Vioxx voluntarily, but rumors of the same problems with other COX-2 inhibitors hit the news, and with the thirty-second news reports, patients stopped taking their medications without consulting their healthcare providers. Wall Street investors unmercifully punished the companies, which lost billions of dollars in market capitalization, drying up new funds for research.

Some of my patients changed from Vioxx to Celebrex. When other Cox-2 inhibitors were implicated, patients stopped taking them. Now, many are back to using the older NSAIDS. Are adverse reactions like gastrointestinal ulceration, bleeding, and death from overdoses follow as we go back to these none-steroidal anti-inflammatory? Most health practitioners will not be surprised. Did patients ask their healthcare providers when considering the trade-off that would result from switching from Cox-2 inhibitors to NSAIDS? Did they consider that switching back to the NSAIDS would increase their risk of death? I doubt it. As the chapter on human social behaviors and herd instincts explains, once the scare starts, rationality will have to wait until the dust settles. Let us add this to other irrational reactions like the Mad Cow disease, Alar in apples and not drinking orange juice due to the anti-carbohydrate craze.

In summary, what is the trade-off? I recommend patients discuss their choices with their healthcare provider. I also like alternatives to medication, like losing weight, using physical therapy, and improving nutrition. People suffering from arthritis should research under the guidance of their prescribing healthcare practitioner, and not make decisions based on a thirty-second news report, a newspaper article, or Internet chat room gossip.

Lack of common sense could lead to rash decisions, which could have worse consequences than the original problem. If you read the *Physician's Desk Reference Guide* about the medications prescribed, you will learn of the hundredths of possible side effects and risks known at the time of FDA approval. Even the samples you receive in the doctor's office contain warning after warning of possible side effects in different clinical situations. After reading all these warnings, you would not take a drug without the assurance of a trusted physician. You will have to assume that your physician has your best interest in mind, and is aware of the possible complications. Let us also think about the assumptions your physician has to make. She has to assume that the pharmaceutical research was scientifically valid and truthful, that the FDA did its job and found the medication safe and effective, and that no further information has emerged of possible risks. She must keep up to date on this information, even with her busy schedule.

You will not find a risk-free medication, nor will you find herbs, vitamins, exercise, or diet programs that do not have risks. If you decide against any of those choices, you will probably be worse off, as many disorders will disable or kill you, if not arrested. Which risks are you willing to take? You will have to select from the options, guided by probabilities and not certainties. The FDA, pharmaceutical companies, physicians, pharmacists, nutritionists, and personal trainers can help you monitor and manage the side effects, but cannot prevent them one hundred percent. Even lawyers cannot prevent adverse effects; risk free treatment does not exist. We need to learn how risks and probabilities work, so we can improve common sense decisions. Risk management should be part of our life decisions, from what treatments to choose, which car to drive, or even what to eat. Too many times, special interest groups and politicians advocate their issues without considering the trade-offs, nor presenting the possible risks.

Most side effects from medications are temporary and mild, but in a small percentage of cases, serious side effects could result in disability or even death. Have you seen the numbers of drug events resulting in significant disability or hospitalization? In the United States, up to one hundred thousand cases per year are reported. I wish the number of patients who would have had adverse reactions or died if no treatment had been prescribed were reported, so we could compare the risks. In addition, they could include and estimate of other known and unknown factors that could be contributing to these statistics. This would be a more balanced way of presenting statistics, but as we tend to advocate in special interest groups, we focus on one side of the coin only. In our adversarial system, other warriors are expected to represent other points of view. As a result, extreme points of view are advocated, none of the parties giving in an inch as it would appear they were capitulating.

In manners of science, we deal with probabilities, not absolutes. If we continue down this path, none of us will take a medication or a prescribed treatment. Some physicians have already stopped delivering babies or dealing with complex medical cases to avoid the adversarial system. Scientific openness, cooperation between different health industries, and trust in your physician will continue to erode. How many pharmaceutical companies will rush to fund studies showing a minimal increase in adverse events in this adversarial environment? If they report these studies, the rash of lawsuits, attacks by consumer advocates, competitors, and media looking for catchy headline stories would have a field day. The executives would lose their jobs, and the scientist who reported the findings would be blackballed from other jobs. Most scientists, physicians, and pharmaceutical executives would have welcomed this information to be better able to understand which patients would benefit most and which were at a higher risk.

Unfortunately, in our adversarial system, there are only two choices—a defective product or not, a company who hid information from the public or not. In reality, we only have one choice: medications that produce side effects and adverse reactions in a percentage of patients, or no medications. The faster we accept this and learn the risks and side effects for a new medication, the better everybody is. Let us stop the negative incentives for companies reporting these findings and be grateful we can make informed decisions. Because science takes time and the frenzy described here when adverse effects are reported is substantial, it is not surprising that company scientists approach findings cautiously, until the weight of evidence confirms reports. Many "positive" results are later found to be chance associations and do not hold up under further study. Even studies having nothing to do with pharmaceutical companies, scientists and physicians disagree on the conclusions of the researchers. If we want to learn and discuss risks or adverse events of a medication, stop special interest groups from activating herd behaviors. There is no free lunch, just a trade-off of risks. If you think pharmaceutical companies should share more of the burden of adverse reactions unknown at the time of approval, discuss the benefits and risks of a system that compensates patients, but do not encourage the adversarial system, which will keep most needed information "sealed" in court papers.

Most people do not understand the medication risks or benefits described in the PDR. In fact, most physicians cannot know, understand, or explain to their patients all the information available on all medications they prescribe, or make a "complete" risk vs. benefits analysis. It is impossible. He will know the most common adverse effects reported, and will try minimizing risk, but he cannot eliminate them. Many books have been written discussing these points. I know this is something we really do not want to hear, especially if we are sick and hoping for help, but it is common sense. We need to accept this and stop incentives that are going in the wrong direction; we need to encourage companies to open their research and not threaten to destroy them, when they do. The adversarial system has encouraged a "cat and mouse game," where for every action there is a reaction, followed by another action by each of the players involved. Trade-offs are not considered. At this time, there is an ambivalent and adversarial relationship between pharmaceutical companies and the public—gratitude towards scientists, executives, and investors who dedicated their lives or money to bring life-saving or enhancing products to the market and the feeling of being ripped off by price gouging or misinformation and undue influence. The pharmaceutical companies have not made their case as to why Americans, who contribute grants and taxes to medical research, have to pay significantly more for the same medications than in other countries. Nor why different companies price similar products at similar prices. Marcia Angell, MD, who presents issues faced by pharmaceutical companies from a more scholarly, academic, and adversarial point of view discusses them in her book, *The Truth about the Drug Companies.*

If the public applies an adversarial system to deal with pharmaceutical companies, expect them to use the same tools. They will have warriors defending their interests, applying the deductive/inductive legalistic approach, in which there are only two choices, theirs, or not theirs. They will not follow the scientific rules, only what is legally required. The adversarial system depends much on deductive and inductive knowledge and not on empirical and scientific knowledge. The public will be the victim of collateral damage. There are so many bright and ethical people in the legal, scientific, political, business, and consumer fields, it is hard to believe they cannot find alternatives for dealing with these issues.

If we require pharmaceutical companies to live by the same rules as businesses—be profitable or perish—expect them to use the marketing tools other business use to thrive. This is an example of using common sense to understand controversial issues. Nobody can have it all!

Elizabeth Wurtzel, with the title of her book, *Prozac Nation*, hit a nerve in our collective consciousness while describing her battle with depression. The concepts I present next, could be applied to other popular medications and treatment options. How did we become a nation in which Prozac, a medication for depression, became a best seller, adorning the front page of our weekly news magazines? The answer has more to do with common sense than the many conspiracy theories brought forward by others. Prozac was the first antidepressant to gain acceptance with general practitioners, not just psychiatrists. Before Prozac, many other antidepressants were available, like Elavil and Pamelor, but the side effects and adverse events were high. Death from an overdose was not a rare event. Primary care physicians and psychiatrists carefully tried low sub-therapeutic doses of these medications, and had poor results. Essentially, older antidepressants were reserved for more severe cases, in which no treatment was riskier than the side effects of the antidepressants.

Then, Prozac was approved. It was the first selective serotonin reuptake inhibitor (SSRI) that the general practitioner could prescribe. It had fewer side effects and lower risk of toxicity or death if an overdose was taken. This enabled people to be treated by their family physician. Ease of use was one of the principal advantages of Prozac, as the initial dose, twenty milligrams, was also the therapeutic or final dose. There was no need to adjust the dosage, which improved the odds of physicians using the medication. With Prozac, this was not a problem—no need to tailor to the individual—opening up the possibilities of treating not just severely depressed patients, but even moderate or mild depressions. Prozac was also found to be effective against some anxiety disorders. More and more physicians and their patients were willing to try Prozac. Celebrities who used Prozac came "out of the closet," and let people know it was "okay" to be depressed; get help, and take Prozac. If they did it, you could, too. Patients requested their physicians to prescribe it for depression, and reported improvement in their depression as well as anxiety or their personalities and social functioning. Some of this anecdotal finding would be later corroborated by research; personality improvement was found to be a consequence of the lessened depression or as other described a bolder attitude. In his best selling book, *Listening to Prozac**, Peter Kramer addressed these issues. The possibility of enhancing our bodies with plastic surgery and our minds with Prozac became a real possibility. I recommend this book as it helps us understand these issues.

The maker of Prozac, Eli Lilly, became the darling of Wall Street, and other pharmaceutical manufacturers rushed to the party with their improved versions of Prozac. This marketing phenomenon is not confined to Prozac; it has happened with cholesterol medications, antibiotics, and even surgical procedures, like the coronary bypass. If you want to learn about the "diffusion of innovation," and how new treatment or medications are incorporated by physicians and the public, I recommend *Diffusion of Innovations*, by Everett M. Rogers.

As more patients were prescribed Prozac, occurrences of side effects, like sexual dysfunction, were found at a higher rate than originally reported. Suicidal thoughts or behaviors were reported. Some practitioners studied these reports and learned to use Prozac as a tool. Prozac was not just a medication. It became the standard for the treating professional whose paradigm included the biological basis of disease and function. The significant improvement that patients experienced on Prozac contributed to the affirmation of their beliefs or methods of practice. Other practitioners, whose treatment paradigm did not include medications, latched onto any reason to attack it. Prozac, the hero, became the villain. Mental health professionals whose paradigm of treatment had not included medication jumped on the Prozac-bashing bandwagon. The war targeted Prozac. Lawsuits accused Prozac of causing violence, suicide, and infanticide. Both sides secured respected experts to be warriors for their point of view.

Let us use common sense. There are millions of mothers all over the world on SSRIs. Rarely, if ever, do they kill their children. So if over 99.99% of mothers on SSRIs do not kill their children, why do special interest groups, whose main agenda is not the protection of children, but the destruction of what Prozac represents, jumped in with these accusations? The reason is that special interest groups with one-tract minds will use whatever information they can to push their agenda, without considering the collateral damage.

While science depends on group trials and uses statistics, comparing and controlling variables before a cause and effect relationship is implied, the legal system and our media are more concerned with individual cases. There are so many known and unknown factors of what affects behaviors; all we can hope for is to use statistics that compare variables. We would need hundreds of cases to know if the behavior correlates to the variable. Scientifically, so many variables cannot be controlled that you could not blame any particular variable, like Prozac, as the cause of the murders. It does not matter which definition of "cause" you use; it would be almost impossible to prove. There are so few cases of mother on medications killing their children, that no significant statistical conclusion could be achieved.

Who would not feel sad about this tragedy? Who would not believe something very wrong happened for a mother to kill her children? Wouldn't we all feel better if we could find a specific reason, a scapegoat on which to blame such behavior so we did not have to deal with other things we could have prevented it? As there is only circumstantial evidence to convict Prozac, it becomes a test of who can convince the jury. The defense will have the advantage if the accused mother can elicit the sympathy of the jury. If the lawyers can get a few jury members who are anti-psychiatry or against medicines and provide experts to testify for them, the probability of winning increases.

The consequences of these decisions and the ensuing publicity will not be considered. If thousands of mothers stop taking their medication, and the rate of infanticide and depression and suicide increases, something else will be blamed. The goal is to win at all costs. If defense lawyers do not use every trick to win, or file for an appeal, they have not done their job. They will not get as many cases if they lose, even if the other side was in the right. We cannot blame the lawyers, however; we who hire them, demand this kind of behavior.

This is not to imply that there are not legitimate cases the court can address, or that a specific case might not need strong advocates. It could take years for evidence to accumulate before science changes its beliefs. As always, a balanced approach is needed, and common sense will help us navigate these transitions. There has been reprehensible behavior by pharmaceutical executives and scientists, who may have willfully hidden information. Some healthcare providers do not keep up with the literature and are callous about their patients' well-being. As in most human endeavors, checks and balances are needed, not an "all or none" approach to problems.

Let us look at how the US Food and Drug Administration (FDA) functions in this adversarial environment. They get it from all directions. The FDA has evolved in the last century. Its role in the first part of the 20th century was to protect us from toxic compounds sold without regard for safety. It was not until the 1960s that Congress added the requirement that pharmaceutical compounds must be safe and effective. Many constituents try influencing the manufacturing, approval, and selling of medications. The FDA is caught between the public who elects government representatives, who then appoint FDA officials, and the pharmaceutical lobbyists who try influencing government representatives. While the public demands safe, risk-free, low cost medications, the lobbyists are trying to protect their industry.

Do you remember the government hearings about US citizens having to go to other countries to get treatment for cancer? The complaints were that the FDA approval process took too long and made companies jump through too many hoops before the American public could buy life saving medications. Senate hearings highlighted ill citizens testifying of the ordeals that had to go thru to get medications at Mexico or Canada, which were not available here. The FDA was accused of delaying the approval of new drugs. Then, the FDA was ordered to develop "fast track" to get the drugs faster in the market. Nervetheless, Congress "forgot" to fund this initiative. Then someone suggested having the pharmaceutical companies pay for those services. So the regulators were been paid by the companies they were to regulate. To complicate things more, the FDA would not match the salaries for drug reviewers offered in the private sector, so they let their reviewers do consulting for the pharmaceutical companies they were reviewing. Now, even if these scientists are very ethical, how can you keep an appearance of impartiality when the reviewers receive payment from the companies they have to review?

Any system as complicated as developing and approving new medications will not run perfectly. Problems will happen, and apparent conflicts of interests will arise, even if none exists. Recently, it was decided that FDA reviewers would no longer be able to consult for the pharmaceutical companies they review, avoiding this conflict of interest. I hope the FDA can figure out how to retain the brightest scientists.

The cycle continues. Now we want to be able to buy our medications in those same countries we did not wanted to buy before, as they are cheaper. Before, we wanted the FDA to approve drugs faster so we did not have to go to those countries, where safety measures might not meet US standards. In an incredible reversal, we now accuse the FDA of approving medications too fast. I am glad I do not have to work for the FDA!

Now let us consider the prescribers of medications. Physicians are frequently criticized for using medications as therapeutic intervention and ignoring other methods of treatment, like vitamins, herbs, exercise, and diet. Never less, most studies in the USA involve medications and not alternative methods of treatment. Why is that?

Common sense will help explain these findings. Insurance companies and the government used to pay for education and research, directly or indirectly, but not anymore. The teaching universities used to provide for independent research and continuing education, but in our penny-wise and pound-foolish "cost control" environment, nobody wants to pay for research or education. The pharmaceutical companies have pick up the tab, even sponsoring consumer education campaigns and informational web pages. Naturally, most of the education and research is related to medications. Would General Motors spend millions on educating us on the benefits of non-automotive transportation? Bicycle makers or consumers' groups who want to decrease pollution or increase mass transportation could spend their money to educate us. Many of the research journals read by physicians are sponsored in part by pharmaceutical companies. They also end up partly sponsoring continuing medical education programs and the annual conventions of many healthcare organizations. A doctor's main tools to treat disease and suffering are medications because nobody is paying for other types of research or education on other treatments. Ultimately the public pays for this research anyway as pharmaceutical companies transfer these cost thru higher medication costs. Before you jump to ask your legislator to stop the pharmaceutical companies from sponsoring most of the education to physicians, be sure funding for continuing education by other agencies is in place. Most pharmaceutical companies are ethical and provide needed education to prescribers, and their influence would be less damaging than no continuing education at all.

Consider the influence of the insurance industry. Obesity is associated with hypertension, diabetes, heart disease, arthritis, and a myriad of other conditions. Health insurance does not pay for the diet or exercise programs that help people lose weight, or for the natural herbs that some studies show to be effective. Now, some insurance companies will cover the cost of an expensive pharmaceutical, like a diet pill, that could have adverse effects. There is no sense in this policy, just decisions made by healthcare and insurance executives many years ago, before we knew what we know about the contributing factors of obesity. Should insurance cover gym memberships or diets, which could save millions of lives and insurance premium dollars on the long run? This apparently simple question opens a myriad of issues. Some of these issues relate to the practice of not considering obesity a disease, and consequently not paying for treatments.

Common sense will help us realize that the present policies are not related to scientific evidence, nor do they make social or economic sense. Do we open Pandora's Box and pay for alternative weight-loss methods? Are other special interest groups, like arthritis groups, going to sue for treatment with shark cartilage? Will it encourage wrongful death class actions suits against insurance companies who refused to pay for gym therapy resulting in cardiac premature deaths? The opening of those floodgates would overwhelm our systems. Already, lawsuits against fast food companies have been filed. This is why change or reversal of policies is so hard. Remember, we all pay through our premiums for what insurance pays in services or lawsuits compensation.

Even in the face of evidence, we know that habits are hard to break, especially those that have served us well in the past. Change requires effort and repetition, and the only companies providing this level of effort are the pharmaceutical companies. They provide journal articles, marketing pieces, continuing education, and regular visits by pharmaceutical representatives with samples to try. They leave coffee mugs, pens, and office articles behind to remind us of their medications and develop brand recognition. To gain physicians' attention and develop goodwill, lunches or dinners are planned away from the office. I am sure, as in all professions, a small percentage of shysters or unscrupulous professionals could be influence wrongly with payouts or trips that serve no educational purpose, but this should be addressed with the particular physician. We are all human. The same marketing tools that work for name recognition, associating good feelings with a product, and brand loyalty, work for medication selection, especially when the differences among medications are minimal. Yet an individual person may have idiosyncratic reactions and respond differently to apparently similar medications. This may represent genetic or environmental factors we are not yet able to recognize. A little common sense explains most of the pharmaceutical companies' behaviors, and shows that they are not part of a conspiracy. They are satisfied with the patients that could be helped by their medication. There are plenty of profits in that plan! They do not need to hide information that their medications could hurt or kill you; they are better off identifying patients that should not take their medications, so physicians do not stop prescribing their medications altogether. If you die, you will not be buying their medications anyway. It is up to us to be sure rules are followed, checks and balances are in place, and incentives are pointing in the right direction. Criminals should be punished swiftly, and if unethical behavior occurs, the perpetrators should be banned from the field.

It takes an average of fifteen years to bring a new medication to market.* Out of 5000 pharmaceutical compounds screened by researchers, only one is approved as a new medicine. From 1980 to 2003, the FDA approved 705 drugs. On average, a new drug costs $800 million to develop and twelve years to be released to the market. Then, pharmaceutical marketers have to educate prescribers on how to use the drug, and why they should try the new medication.

How about adverse effects discovered as medications are exposed to millions of people? It is very difficult to recruit patients that fulfill a specific profile. Only a few patients will qualify for or complete the research protocol. However, when the drug is approved, it is available to millions of patients, even those with complicating factors excluded from the original approval studies. Serious side effects missed in the original studies could appear.

Take a hypothetical example. To get approval from the FDA, drug A, was studied in 20,000 patients. During the testing, all the symptoms the patients suffered were reported, from sore throats to fever, nausea, or itching. Many symptoms could be caused by allergies or a cold, or other factors not related to the drug we are investigating, but they need to be reported anyway, as the researches are doing double blind studies, and cannot tell if somebody is taking the active medication or a placebo. At the end, researchers run a statistical analysis to see if the rate of sore throat or fever or heart attacks were statistically significant in the people who took the medication or if such affects occurred at the same rate as those who took the sugar pill. Many times, they are not.

Then drug A is prescribed to 100,000 people, and as they live in the real world, these patients may have a "little" high blood pressure, diabetes, or underlying cardiac disease that neither they nor their doctors knew they had. They may drink alcohol and smoke. To get drug A approved during research, they had to control and avoid these variables to see if the drug was effective and not confuse the findings with situations presented by different patients with other complications. Now, as millions of "real world patients" are exposed to the new medication, reports of heart attacks or fever may rise. In the initial studies, there may have been ten reported heart attacks in the 10,000 patients who took the new medication and nine in the placebo group. Statistical analysis will probably show no difference between these two groups; it was just chance that there was one extra heart attack in the medicated group. However, as 100,000 "complicated" patients take the medication; two hundred people have a heart attack. That is more than expected, (10/10,000 in the initial studies, which translates to

100/100,000, later). At two hundred heart attacks, the effect is double what was expected. This statistic will be reported as "doubling your risk of heart attack."

In reality, all that means is that during the experiment for FDA approval, only one patient out of 1,000 suffered a heart attack. As 100,000 new patients, who probably had other factors influencing their rate of heart attacks, take the medication, 2 out of 1,000 patients have one. So 998 out of a thousand will not have a hearth attack. Assuming this medication is helping them and may be better than other available treatments, why should it be taken off the market? People can decide if they want to take the risk or not.

If you were a scientist working for the pharmaceutical company, and see these reports, would you pull it before you could design and complete studies to see if there was really an increase or if it was just a chance association? What if it only happened to people with previous heart conditions? Would you keep 999 people from getting relief to their problem to avoid one extra possible heart attack? If you are one of those 999 getting relief, do you want a choice?

People will answer these questions differently. There must be a better way to handle these problems. Most people would want to know what type of patients with what kind of complications suffered heart attacks, or if duration of exposure increased the risk. Unfortunately, the cat and mouse game starts even before the lawsuits are filed. One side tries to prove there was deception from the beginning, that the pharmaceutical companies hid reports of adverse effects.

The pharmaceutical companies will take the opposite adversarial position. They could have been trying to minimize bad publicity until more evidence was available. This would avoid taking the product off the shelves or informing doctors of the ongoing study, as perhaps it was just a chance association. They could be trying to identify which patients should avoid the new medication. But perhaps a certain scientist or executive knew of the risks, but minimized them so their product would sell well and be established as the "gold standard" before the negative publicity got out. Whatever the reason, the moment they admit there might be patients who could suffer adverse effects, lawsuits will follow, and the "herd mentality" will follow.

Let us throw into the brew the wishes and expectations of the shareholders of the pharmaceutical companies, who have invested millions of dollars and expect a return. Add human folly, bad luck, manufacturing problems, and competition from other companies. Other nations may not respect patents and produce pirated products. So many things can go wrong!

When you think about it, taking that little pill is almost an act of faith. Not only do you have to have faith that the pharmaceutical company did not lie about its research findings to the FDA, but also that it was manufactured correctly, and that it contains the proper compound at the right doses. Your physician had to make the right diagnosis and select the right treatment. You have to trust that the pharmacist gave you the right medication, and then you have to hope you are not the one in 10,000 that develops an allergic reaction or suffers an adverse effect. Maybe sweating at the gym or saying no to desert is not such a sacrifice. On the other hand, is it? Take a survey at the mall. Would you prefer to sweat at the gym and give up desserts, or take a pill every morning to control your weight?

Human nature affects how we deal with the issues. The search for security, certainty, and the easy way out, is at the root of some of these problems. We live in a very threatening world. We might not need to fight tigers, but we are faced with muggers, terrorists, human folly, and disease. We even risk adverse reactions if we take medication. No matter how many things we consider, we still have to answer the question, "Do I, or do I not take the medication?" In matters of science, there is no certainty. Here, the "virtue of doubt" is necessary.

An article about Alan Greenspan, written by Robert J. Samuelson in my local newspaper, reported that Alan Greenspan had been the chairperson of the Federal Reserve Board for the past eighteen years, and was one of the world's most influential economists. Some consider him the greatest central banker, who, through different administrations, was able to juggle all kinds of threats to the economy. From Mr. Samuelson's article, come these quote:

"A second principle is the inevitability of ignorance. The *economy* is so complex and changes so rapidly that no *economic* model—"no matter how detailed or how well conceived," he told the conference, "can ever capture reality." This explains Greenspan's dourness: the certainty of uncertainty."

Now substitute "Life" or "Human Nature" for the word "economy" and read it again.

CHAPTER NINE

CONSERVATIVES VS. LIBERALS

"You can check out any time you want,
but you can never leave."
—The Eagles, "Hotel California"

I remember watching Bill O' Reilly's interview of President George W. Bush before the 2004 election. They were unable to explain why Hollywood is so liberal. I think I have an answer. The short version is that the strength of traits that serves the entertainer well is what also leads people toward the Liberal approach as shown in the table below. The process of common sense applied to the information presented in this book will clarify the answer. We have genetic predispositions that help us adjust to our environment. There are limited homeostatic adjustments that our organism can apply to improve the odds of survival. Our cognitive-behavioral patterns and the mode of thinking we use most are shaped by our underlying cognitive strengths. Our stable, but modifiable, personalities filter the information we receive and send. Birth order can be a powerful factor. The social moods of the times also influence us, as they represent the aggregate sum of all of society's individual interactions. The power of the group can take us where we would never go on our own, to our advantage or disadvantage. Human nature, religion, and politics are

125

learned from our families and surrounding culture, influencing whether we are more likely to be liberal or conservative. That is why intelligent, educated, and well-intentioned people given the same facts can arrive at different conclusions or come up with different ways to deal with problems. Look at table C-L, in which I have summarized the primary differences between conservatives and liberals.

Table Conservative/Liberal

Conservatives	Liberals
Power diffused in local governments (split)	Strong central power (whole)
Individual is the center	Group politics
Concerned with cost vs. benefit analysis	In principle, environment, society first, analysis secondary
Traditional, incremental changes (Risk/harm avoidance-high)	Theoretical, wholesale changes (Risk/harm avoidance low)
Reserved in emotional displays	Expressive in emotional displays
Frugal in economic matters (Low novelty seeking)	Thrifty in economic matters (High novelty seeking)
Determination, perfectionist, rule follower (High perseverance)	Rules can be interpreted differently or easily changed if necessary (Low perseverance)
Independent, people's feeling need not interfere with the facts or rules (Low reward dependence)	Sociable, sympathetic, sentimental (High reward dependence)

These are the traits usually described in the media. They represent degrees, not extremes. In parentheses are the personality and right- and left-brain hemisphere traits that mirror qualities usually identified by the media. There are similarities between the qualities found in the left and right hemispheres of the brain and those described as conservative vs. liberal. Maybe that is why businesspersons tend to be conservative, and entertainment professionals tend to be liberal. To entertain, you need to form a connection with your public, and emotions get immediate results. The moment you lose your emotional connection, your success as an entertainer diminishes. In business, developing long-term plans takes precedence over our emotions, rewarding those who can control their emotions and maintain a course of action, even when other people's feelings get hurt. The percentage of personality traits an individual has will also influence whether that person is more likely to be liberal or conservative as explained in the differences in between the accountant and the actor's personality.

If an office receptionist falls ill and cannot perform his job, the business still needs someone to make appointments, manage the phone, and take messages. An office manager can separate the tasks, assign them to others, or hire someone new. From an emotional point of view (the liberal view), the feelings and needs of the ill employee take center stage. The policies and procedures of the company will be secondary. The manager, the company, or the courts can change or reinterpret the rules.

From a conservative point of view (and their tragic view of life), people get sick, and policies and procedures are in place to deal with the problems. These policies are followed to the letter, no matter the consequences. It would not be fair to change the rules for an individual, as other employees would pay a price (like extra work), plus everybody would expect the rules to be changed for them.

I imagine readers taking sides and adding more arguments to validate their points of view. Liberals, with their positive view of human nature, may call the conservative executive heartless. If a customer or coworker complains, they expect understanding of the dilemma caused by the ill employee.

The conservative, rationally and objectively, will consider the advantages and disadvantages of different solutions. They prioritize getting the job done understanding that no matter what decision is taken some will suffer.

In most cases, compromises are found. Depending on how large the business is, laws to protect workers are in place. Nevertheless, no matter how many laws or regulations, human judgment will always be involved.

Some people try to apply the legal system to resolve every problem, but the legal system has a different way of acquiring and applying knowledge. One of the books that inspired me to write about common sense was, *The Death of Common Sense*, by Howard Phillips. He addresses the historical, political, and social developments that contributed to the death of common sense in the legal system. In example after example, he shows that we will never be able to eliminate the need for common sense, as we cannot pass enough laws or regulations to cover every facet of human interaction. We cannot predict Real life, variables, known and unknown cannot be anticipated. Bureaucracies grow, regulations multiply, and nobody can keep up with them. We need to hire warriors (lawyers) and experts to understand their requirements. When was the last time you tried figuring out the tax code? I strongly recommend the writings of Thomas Sowell* who eloquently explained many of the concepts I presented in this chapter and influenced me with his writings.

There are different points of view of the nature of man, and the conservative and liberal views are very different. The conservative view could be the "tragic view of life." No matter what we do to improve society, there will be suffering. People will get sick, suffer accidents, and die. Because of man's selfish nature, if he is left to his own devices, without the checks and balances of constitutional democracies, he will enslave or destroy others, and ultimately, himself. This concept is similar to the "original sin" doctrine, in which we are all born sinners, and only through the grace of God, *not man*, can man be saved. This is significant difference between conservatives and liberals and one reason these groups cannot understand each other. Liberals see humans as having been born with a "blank slate," without predispositions to selfishness. It is society, the powerful or the economic system that corrupts man, as many times they still follow the Nobel Savage conception of Human Nature. Their thinking style is *idealistic*, and they tend to be high in *reward dependence*. Because of these characteristics, they believe the educated or "enlightened," will guide man, without needing God to redeem or save him. Emotions take a more central role than adherence to social, political, or religious rules. This encourages artistic forms of expression, in which even outrageous forms of behavior are tolerated.

Conservatives believe man is born with a tendency to be selfish, in matters of sex and social positioning, that unless man is controlled, everyone will suffer. Because of these beliefs, conservatives tend to bring God to public policy. He will have more left hemisphere characteristics, liking law and order, believing rules are developed for the good of all and emotional expressions are not tolerated. While the liberal will quickly change their plan course of action and help

129

people who are suffering, the conservative assumes suffering is part of life, and tries keeping emotions in check while rationally planning how to help and considering the consequences of their help. In different situations, one approach may be more effective than the other is, or as frequently happens, a compromise occurs. The two groups cannot agree on the problem or ways to improve it.

Reading the United States Constitution and the writings of the founding fathers, the "tragic view of life," appears to have had a more significant influence. From the checks and balances between the executive, legislative, and judicial branches of government to the understanding of the fragility of the document. They understood that even if power could corrupt us, we would still have to govern each other. Amendments like the Bill of Rights were added to prevent the "natural" human tendency to nepotism, corruption, and silencing of dissent. That is another reason why conservatives are tough on crime. Liberals want to rehabilitate or make up for what caused the criminal lifestyle. Liberals start with the premise that man is good and lack of education or opportunity corrupts him. Conservatives believe all humans are born with drives and passions that cannot be controlled or prevented by education or rehabilitation. This is why conservatives need God to help control their drives and redeem them, and liberals do not.

Scientific knowledge points to the corroboration of the conservative view of human nature; we are driven by instincts, powerful, illogical emotions, unconscious crowd behavior, and our life experiences. We cannot turn our backs on these facts and hope that law, reeducation, or wishful thinking, will return us to the state of the noble savage, which never existed. Religious concepts like been born with original sin, can be understood also from the tragic view of life approach, or even science. That is why wishful and youthful rejections of traditional morality or religion in the name of modern-day science is mistaken. These principles, has guided civilization for thousands of years. This knowledge was acquired and transmitted by our ancestors, who often paid with their lives so that we could enjoy the fruit of their efforts. Be it with the wisdom of religious or spiritual mechanisms, science, philosophy, or law, we have sufficient checks and balances to help us move forward, but only after considering the tradeoffs of our decisions, and how it fits, or not, with the wisdom of the ages. Denial will not change human nature, but careful study and understanding will help us modulate its possible consequences and encourage its positive aspects. Our outdated, selfish genes will cause much trouble if not managed properly. Whether you are religious or secularist, the passions and urges we all experience could destroy us. Avoiding situations in which our outdated urges thrive will help the journey. As the rock band, The Eagles, in their song "Hotel California" better express it, "You can checkout anytime you want, but you can never leave." You can try avoiding reality, but you cannot escape it. Most of the scientific knowledge or spiritual insights we have acquired fit into our schemes of things as long as we do not built a rigid wall around them. Einstein's theories help explain phenomenon that could not be understood with previous views of the world, and they did not result in wholesale discrediting of Newton's theories. As it was hard for scientists who had spent their lives believing the old theories to change their beliefs, it will be hard for us to change our views of the world. Sometimes we will have to admit we were wrong and review our conclusions and beliefs. This is an ongoing challenge for everyone. Common sense will help you through this mountain of information.

The same way we need both halves of our brain to function best, we also need conservative and liberal points of view. Balancing our needs requires constant vigilance and effort, without letting emotions or rationality completely dominate. If only one aspect were needed, we would have evolved, or would have been created, that way, with mainly R or L Brain Hemisphere strengths.

The liberal establishment needs to reassess and develop a theory and practice of government that takes into account recent findings regarding human nature. If not, their core constituents in the United States will continue to dwindle. Their leaders continue to advocate solutions based on old theories discarded by most voters. We could lose those checks and balances that foster our ability to change. People's emotional and relationship needs and creativity could be diminished. Group politics and special interest groups continue to divide us. This encouragement of the "parts," and not the "whole," goes against what the liberals represent best.

Conservatives need to reassess their concept of the ghost in the machine, and incorporate new scientific findings that explain how the mind and the body are of the same essence. The concept of the Soul could encompass many of the qualities that traditionally have been ascribed to the mind. Conservatives, as well as liberals, should study and understand how the characteristics we once thought belonged to the soul, may be influenced by the mind and brain, which are of the same essence as the body. Conservative points of view are increasing in public policy, but they need to modulate their frustration with the rate of change in the courts. Overturning previous court decisions is hard, as it should be. In social policies, no matter how strongly we believe in the need to overturn a Supreme Court decision, we need to first help others see and agree with the reasons for the change. If you are able to easily reverse or change court decisions, the other camp can do it to you, also. History shows that conservative and liberal approaches cycle, and the other camp, if not in agreement with you, could reverse the decision. Unfortunately, court decisions wrong by most moral or constitutional standards may take a long time to reverse. This is the price of a constitutional democracy.

Ms. Conservative, Mr. Liberal, please consider the information in this book and stop calling each other names. You have different conceptions of human nature, different strengths, personality traits, and experiences. If our bodies function best with two brain hemispheres, two hands, eyes, feet, and chromosomes, why can't we function as liberals and conservatives? In different situations or times, some traits will dominate, but always with the check and balances of the other characteristics.

If self-reliance and personal responsibility continue to erode, we will abdicate our liberties and responsibilities to special interest groups that wait for opportunities to impose their ways.

By now, you have probably figured out why the mental health field tends to be more liberal than other professions are. You need a more active right hemisphere, where relationships and emotional difficulties are understood and handled easily. You need strong "rewards-dependent" personality traits, where your personal satisfaction comes from helping others, not from corporate spreadsheets or balancing a budget.

An important trait is the ability to work with all types of emotional, cognitive, and behavioral dysfunctions, which could be disturbing to many people. It is often necessary to help the whole person, not just a particular problem; we may need to tolerate some disturbing behaviors while we help the whole person change those behaviors. Teachers, who maintained an idealistic view of how much man could help man, often influenced mental health professionals. As there was not much known about the causes or effective treatments of some disorders, the emphasis, for a while, was to take a socio-political approach, especially for cases like schizophrenia. As the burden of caring for these patients was significant, and many times not covered by health insurance, the therapist became the activist advocating for more government help. A more liberal concept—government involved in your lives. The fact that we are trying to help people through talk or medication increases our sense that humans can help change humans, and may make some religious leaders that completely depend on God for healing, uncomfortable. It is up to us to explain to them how our services are complementary and not mutually exclusive. We in the mental health fields have to understand how working as a special interest group may interfere with our ability to understand and be effective in matters of public policy. We need to stop calling people ignorant or accusing them of being prejudiced; we should look in the mirror first. We need a return to common sense and the acceptance that nothing is certain. We need to stop the public battles that contribute to the public's confusion and workout our professional differences in a scholarly fashion. While our personal views on politics, philosophy, and religion may color our approach, it should not interfere with our professional consensus, or the way we handle problems. As a profession, we have done a poor job of separating our personal views from our professional duties. This is a free country, and you can express whatever ideas you have, but as a licensed professional, you are expected to comply with the community or national standards of your licensing board.

Too many times, the mental health professional forgets that we all function better when both sides of our brain and all personality traits are considered. Attacks on scientific reductionism are often misplaced and misguided. When science is understood and used properly, it only reduces the suffering of the patient and his family. I repeat what Dr. Guze so eloquently said:

> Nothing can be more truly humanitarian than working for and applying effective knowledge to prevent or ameliorate human suffering. Approaches that are compassionate but ineffective many times help more assuage our feelings of doing something than helping patients.

Read these two sentences again. This lesson could prevent much suffering and waste of resources. The scientific method has played a significant part in the progress of Western culture and its contributions to the world. Even though American medicine may have issues to resolve, it is still top-notch, and people from all over the world come to America for treatment or training. Those who cannot afford to come to the US read journals and textbooks and benefit from our research. The fact that some Americans do not have access to this system is not the fault of science or medicine, but of sociopolitical and economic forces. Can medicine benefit from a more humane touch? Sure. Can mental health professions benefit from applying scientific principles? Definitely.

Conclusions

I have tried to present the importance of not forgetting our beloved friend, Common Sense. I have used examples from medicine, science, and psychiatry. However, the concepts I presented here, could be applied in most fields of knowledge. I have not contributed any new findings, just tried to simplify and connect what other authors have presented after spending years of their lives on these studies. Again, I ask for their forgiveness if I simplify too much or misinterpret their findings.

In summary:

- The knowledge base has exploded exponentially and its distribution improved significantly since the advent of the Internet.
- Practitioners need to become experts in narrow fields, as nobody can keep up with the magnitude of knowledge available.
- Experts tend to form organizations that require the development of specialized language, styles of thinking, and culture, with agreed rules of acquiring and disseminating knowledge.
- Special interest groups have developed to lobby and advocate for their special interest.
- The non-expert must try to integrate this specialty knowledge with the rest of his knowledge.

- No expert or special interest group can give us more than an approximation of reality.
- Common sense is sound judgment acquired through judicious observation and interaction with our environment, in combination with our abilities to intuit.
- We are all born with the ability to use and grow our common sense.
- Both formal and informal education raises our level of common sense.
- Multiple factors influence how we perceive the issues or problems and develop common sense:
  - A. Styles of Thinking
  - B. Ways of acquiring knowledge
  - C. Genetic and psycho-neurological endowment
  - D. Familial Influences
  - E. Life experiences
  - F. Our tendency to follow the crowd
  - G. Personality traits
  - H. Assumptions of human nature
  - I. Prior knowledge
  - J. Religious, ethical, moral beliefs
  - K. How hard are we willing to work at acquiring it.

- The adversarial system has encroached on our daily discourses, fostering personal resentment, not the resolution of issues.

Common sense will help you integrate this information and help you be generally right and avoid being precisely wrong.

Appendix I

The Adversarial System

"We are not enemies, but friends. We must not be enemies. Though passion may have strained, it must not break our bonds of affection. The mystic chords of memory, stretching from every battlefield and patriot's grave to every living heart and hearthstone all over this broad land will yet swell the chorus of the Union, when again touched, as surely they will be, by the better angels of our nature."

Abraham Lincoln

Many writers trace the adversarial system to the Middle Ages. Parties resolved disputes by a duel, or hired accomplish combatants to represent them. In Western Europe, this approach was identified as "judicious Dei," (The judgment of God). It was assumed that God would strengthen the arm of the combatant in the right, who would consequently win. This systems evolved into system were two opposing views fight it out and one winner emerges. Because there can only be one winner, both sides have a "winner takes all" approach. They will not only attack the facts and arguments of the other side, but will mount personal attacks on the other combatant. This ultimately causes resentments and bitterness, by not only the loser, but also the winner, who emerges weakened by the contest. At the end of the battle, one side does not concede that the other side won because they were in the right, but accuses the winner of cheating, lying, or manipulating the public or jury. Instead of cooperating with the verdict, the sabotaging and personal attacks intensify. This system prevents us from finding the truth or encouraging the other side to understand and maybe change their point of view. There are only two options, win or lose.

We could try other systems, such as accepting the proposals on which most agree, or compromise, so that every "combatant" gives up something to gain something, but this is harder than just destroying your opponent. It will always be easier to destroy than construct, and we will always take the easy way out. How many politicians, TV and radio pundits, or even ourselves are willing to spend the time and effort to listen to all aspects of an argument, consider the trade-offs, and adjust our point of view? I have heard more people apologize for doing something wrong than defenders of positions going public and reporting changes of opinion. I have seen opposing forces screaming at each other, but never had the pleasure of commentators trying to find a compromise. It only polarizes the public's viewpoints. Could producers add a third point of view, or have debaters spending five minutes trying to find common ground? How about spending time helping us understand why people with similar backgrounds and goals, using the same facts, can arrive at such different conclusions?

In the past few years, practically every presidential election in the United States has been between two candidates with opposite points of view and is decided by only a few percentage points, between 49% and 51%. The polarization continues, even when attacked by an enemy that calls for destruction of our way of life. Is it an artifact of our bi-partisan practices, or just another example of binary thinking? If we do not heed President Lincoln's words, we will repeat the same mistakes and pay again with blood, sweat, and tears. The enemy does not need to defeat us, just instill enough doubt and keep us fighting within ourselves, to render us impotent. Divide and conquer—even children know this strategy, why do politicians not?

I do not want to suppress dissension or discussion, but the adversarial system will only encourage terrorists. If children can take the disagreements of their parents and use them to get what they want, imagine what the terrorists can do. Paraphrasing Yogi Berra, its déjà vu all over again.

Consilience

Consilience is "knowledge that will connect all fields," which has a strong attraction for most people. This could cloud our common sense if we prematurely think science has already provided the answer.

I recommend *Consilience*,* by EO Wilson, which elegantly explains the concept. John Hogan's book, *The End of Science*,* also addresses many of these questions. The idea is that the time will come that, as knowledge expands, a set of rules or formulas will explain all phenomena and see the connections between fields as diverse as the social and physical sciences. Scientists and philosophers throughout the centuries have tried to express similar concepts. In religion, for example, God has been the common denominator that "explains it all." Deists see nature as the essence of God. Scientists are in search of the formula or theory that will unite all sciences and explain everything. This is an example of how common sense can help you with "unknown" or difficult concepts and not prematurely assume that we have found it. Led Zeppelin, a popular rock band, struck a cord with their song, "Stairway to Heaven." Listen carefully as it builds to its climax, the last verse. Like any work of art, it is open to subjective interpretation. It has elements of many of the concepts I have discussed. I will tell you my interpretation, and include in parenthesis the words of the last paragraph of the song, so that you may derive your own conclusions.

From the "mean genes"/sinful nature (*our shadows larger than our soul*)

To the search of knowledge/salvation through "old" philosophy, science, religion (*there is an old lady we all know*)

providing enlightenment (*who shines white light*)

And turning all to gold, the timeless symbol of immutable value and security (*wanting to show how everything still turns to gold*)

Searching for the way and answers (*and if you listen very hard, the tune will come to you at last*)

And a popular conception of consilience (*where all is one and one is all*)

Nevertheless, each individual trying to buy security/immortality even after listening to the tune (*and she is buying a stairway to haven*).

Our old lady, Ms. Common Sense, comes to the rescue. She will not give us the answer to our questions or explain behaviors, but she will help us integrate forms of knowledge and come up with "on-going, working solutions" that integrate religion, morals, biology, development, and other factors in a reasonable, "all is one, one is all" way.

Common Thinking Tendencies*

1. Binary thinking – We think in opposites. In early childhood, one of the first things we learn is "mine," as opposed to "yours," and "no," as opposed to "yes."

2. When faced with many options, we tend to become confused and indecisive.

3. We tend to think opposites are true. If you prove somebody "wrong," it does not mean you are "right."

4. We are comfortable with familiarity. We explore what we already know.

5. If we are content with a given solution, we are less likely to consider alternatives.

6. When we have made up our minds, we tend to look for evidence that reinforces our decision and does not contradict it.

7. Once we settle an issue in our minds, we review other concepts from this perception of truth, and build on that issue without reconsidering it.

8. Proving something "wrong" is much easier than proving something "right." That is why we criticize and destroy, instead of building.

9. Knowledge is about the past. Thinking is about the future.

10. We sound very good when we analyze a situation the facts of which we already know. (This is like Monday-night quarterbacking.)

Useful communication must always be in the language of the receiver. Non-experts are not stupid, ignorant, or lazy. They just do not understand your language.

Appendix II

Common Sense in Times of War

At the time of this writing, we are involved in a crisis; the tiger is coming to devour us, and we are fighting back. In times like this, we need strong leaders to make tough decisions that could mean life or death for some, or cause significant changes of the principles by which we live. This requires a degree of expertise most of us do not have, and for experts to exchange knowledge and opinions before our leader can decide a course of action. The president needs to process information and advice that, at times, is contradictory. He needs to juggle special interest group and deal with the inevitable mistakes. He needs to be involved in the running of the federal government, selecting Supreme Court nominees that will influence our country for years to come, providing disaster relief leadership, and influencing where our tax money will be spent over the next few years. In addition, he still needs to be a parent, a spouse, and care for their own needs. The constant barrage of personal attacks that our leaders are subjected to on a daily basis is overwhelming! I am torn between thinking these people are ruthless politicians or that they are citizens willing to sink the country to maintain or come to power. Maybe they missed Psychology 101 in college, or maybe they are so driven by emotion, that their rational cortex has not yet taken over. Perhaps they have such different beliefs and are so used to the adversarial system that they can not adjust or hold their anger about a particular issue. Terrorists, who want our destruction, read and listen to the same reports. The personal attacks only encourage our enemies and provide ammunition to justify their slaughter. Stop fighting the last war; this is not Vietnam. This war is being fought on many fronts, and already long-term allies are throwing punches at each other. We need to avoid a war of ideas and find common ground in what unites us, as President Lincoln expressed so well in the Gettysburg Address.

THE GETTYSBURG ADDRESS
NOVEMBER 19, 1863

Four score and seven years ago our fathers brought forth on this continent, a new nation, conceived in liberty, and dedicated to the proposition that all men are created equal.

Now we are engaged in a great civil war, testing whether that nation, or any nation so conceived and so dedicated, can long endure. We are met on a great battlefield of that war. We have come to dedicate a portion of that field, as a final resting-place for those who here gave their lives that this nation might live. It is altogether fitting and proper that we should do this.

But, in a larger sense, we cannot dedicate...we cannot consecrate...we cannot hallow...this ground. The brave men, living and dead, who struggled here, have consecrated it far above our poor power to add or detract. The world will little note nor long remember what we say here, but it can never forget what they did here. It is for us, the living, rather, to be dedicated here to the unfinished work which they who fought here have thus far so nobly advanced. It is rather for us to be here dedicated to the great task remaining before us...that from these honored dead we take increased devotion to that cause for which they gave the last measure of devotion; that we here highly resolve that these dead shall not have died in vain; that this nation, under God, shall have a new birth of freedom; and that government of the people, by the people, for the people, shall not perish from the earth.

Abraham Lincoln

I can see president Lincoln, standing tall by our soldiers grave or by the World Trade Center reminding us that these shall not have died in vain, while by his side, president Reagan encourages the Terrorist to "bring down the wall," the terrorist fear mongering wall, that tries to prevent the exchange of ideas.

Bibliography

Angell, Marcia. *The Truth about the Drug Companies*. Random House, 2004.

Basler, Roy P., ed. *The Collected Works of Abraham Lincoln*.

Bernstein, Peter L. *Against the Gods, the Remarkable Story of Risk*. 1996.

Berreby, David. *Us and Them*. Little Brown and Company, 2005.

Bronowski, J. *The Common Sense of Science*. 1951.

Burnham, Terry, and Jay Phelan. *Mean Genes: From Sex to Money to Food: Taming Our Primal Instincts*. Penguin Books, 2001.

Carter, Stephen L. *Civility, Manners, Morals, and the Etiquette of Democracy*. Basic Books, 1998.

Clonninger, C. Robert. *Feeling Good: The Science of Well Being*. John Wiley & Sons, Inc., 2004

Conley, Dalton. *The Pecking Order: Which Siblings Succeed and Why*. Pantheon Books, 2004.

Coren, Stanley. *The Left-Hander Syndrome*. Vintage Books, 1993.

Damasio, Antonio. *Looking for Spinoza: Joy, Sorrow, and the Feeling Brain*. Harcourt Books, 2003.

——. *Descartes' Error: Emotion, Reason, and the Human Brain*. G.P. Putnam's Sons, 1994.

Dawkins, Richard. *The Selfish Gene*. The Oxford Press, Inc.

DeBono, Edward. *De Bono's Thinking Course: Facts on File.* 1994.

Diagnostic Criteria from the Diagnostic and Statistical Manual: IV-TR. The American Psychiatric Association, Washington D.C., 2000.

Glasser, William. *Warning: Psychiatry Can Be Hazardous to Your Mental Health.* HarperCollins Publishing Inc., 2003.

Goldberg, Elkhonon. *The Wisdom Paradox.* Penguin Group, USA, 2005.

Goodwin, Donald W., and Samuel B. Guze. *Psychiatric Diagnosis.* Oxford University Press.

Guze, Samuel B. *Why Psychiatry is a Branch of Medicine.* The Oxford University Press, Inc., 1992.

Harrison, Allen F., and Robert M. Bramson. *Styles of Thinking, Strategies for Asking Questions, Making Decisions, and Solving Problems.* 1982.

Hawkins, Stephen, and Leonard Mlodinow. *A Briefer History of Time.* Bantam Books, Oct 2005.

Hoff-Sommers, Christina, and Sally Satel. *One Nation Under Therapy: How the Helping Culture Is Eroding Self-Reliance.* St. Martin's Press, 2005.

Horgan, John. *The End of Science, Facing the Limits of Knowledge in the Twilight of the Scientific Age.* Helix Books, 1996.

Howard, Phillip K. *The Death of Common Sense.* Random House, Inc. Anchor Press Edition. Vintage Book, 1994.

Isaac, Rachel J., and Virginia C Armat. *Madness in the Streets: How Psychiatry and the Law Abandoned the Men tally Ill.*

Kandal, Eric. *Principles of Neural Science.* Fourth edition, 2000.

Kramer, Peter D. *Listening to Prozac.* Viking Press, 1993.

Lidz, Charles W., et al. *Informed Consent.* The Guildford

Press, NY, 1984.
Mackay, Charles. *Extraordinary Popular Delusions and the Madness of Crowds.* Harmony Books, NY, NY, 1980.
McNeill, Daniel, and Paul Freiberger. *Fuzzy Logic.* First Touchstone Edition, 1994.
Prechter, Robert R. *The Wave Principle of Human Social Behavior and the New Science of Socionomics.* New Classics Library, 1999.
Pinker, Steven. *The Blank Slate: The Modern Denial of Human Nature.* Penguin Books, Ltd., 2002.
The Paradox Principle. Price Waterhouse Change Integration Team.
Ratey, John J. *A User's Guide to the Brain.* First Vintage Books Edition, Jan 2002.
Rogers, Everett M. *Diffusion of Innovations.* The Free Press, Div. Simon and Schuster, Inc., NY, NY, 1983.
Schlesinger, Arthur M. *The Disuniting of America: Reflections on a Multicultural Society.* Norton edition, 1992.
Sowell, Thomas. *The Vision of the Anointed: Self-Congratulation as a Basis for Social Sciences.* Basic Books, a division of HarperCollins Publishers, 1995.
Sulloway, Frank J. *Born to Rebel: Birth Order, Family Dynamics, and Creative Lives.* Pantheon Books, 1996.
The Great Courses. The Teaching Company, 1-800-TEACH-12.
Zarefsky, David. *Argumentation: The Study of Effective Reasoning.* 2001.

Notes and Other References*

Preface—The Return of Common Sense—adapted from an anonymous report on the Internet, "A Eulogy for Common Sense."

The challenge is to be broadly right and not precisely wrong—From the Price Waterhouse team.

If you cannot find the source for topics discussed in this book, please contact me via e-mail.

"Common Thinking Tools" inspired by Thomas Sowell.

"Judicious Dei" information obtained from multiple sources on the Internet and DeBono's book.

Due to the changeable nature of the World Wide Web, I have not included Internet addresses for articles I have used. Please do your own careful research. I will keep as current a list of resources as possible on my Web site: commonsense-mentalhealth.com.

You will be able to join others in discussion rooms about the concepts presented in this book and can subscribe to our monthly newsletter.

Web address: www.commonsense-mentalhealth.com

E-mail:TROCS@commonsense-mentalhealth.com

Behavioral Healthcare Solutions

Behavioral health problems represent some of the most complex and least understood of all healthcare issues. For every strong advocate of a particular view or paradigm, many others see the issues differently. This has contributed to much confusion and bewilderment when trying to access care or get answers to basic healthcare issues. That is why our logo is the gyroscope, a device whose movements are a synthesis of competing forces. It can move along a string or rotate on a pinhead while the rings spin in all directions. It mirrors the paradox we face in behavioral healthcare today.

Let our company help you understand and manage these paradoxes so you can achieve your goals. The challenge is to be broadly right and avoid being precisely wrong. We bring extensive experience and after listening to your needs, we are able to present you with a variety of suggestions, enabling you to select the best course of action for your enterprise. Our commitment is to give you common sense answers to your questions and needs. We are able to give you support, as well. Give us a call so we can find the answers you need.

Fax: 1-904-296-3144

E-mail- drtoro@bellsouth.net

www.bhnc.yourmd.com